Content

I0481814

Ketogenic Diet Salad Recipes

Trying out a new diet can be difficult. You have to avoid some foods and eat more of others. It also means you need to buy new ingredients. The process can be physically draining. But you can try out the ketogenic diet. This diet has some simple and tasty salad recipes to keep you fit and healthy.

The ketogenic diet promotes weight loss by putting the body in the ketosis state. This state allows dieters to use fat as energy. In this metabolic state, fat is the source of energy rather than glucose. Ketones are produced when a person enters this metabolic state and the body as an auxiliary source of power uses it.

Burning fat is one of many benefits that ketosis offers. Some other benefits include fewer cravings, more self-control, lower caloric intake and more physical activity. Keto dieters experience and overall improvement in their health and have increased energy levels for mental and physical activities.

Being on a keto diet doesn't have to be difficult. Whether you started dieting a while ago or you just joined the train, you can find something tasty to keep you going. Most people are shocked when they discover that the keto diet has a wide range of foods for every occasion. You can have snacks, food, drinks, desserts and even salads that are not just great looking but tasty as well.

This eBook contains the best salad recipes for every occasion. They are simple and the ingredients can be gotten without a hassle. It contains salads with fruits, vegetables, meat, chicken, fish and more.

There is nothing tastier than low carb keto salads. It doesn't matter if you are having them alone or for dinner or lunch. Enjoy our sweet keto salads in every season.

1. BLUE CHEESE COLESLAW

Preparation time 15 minutes

Calories 340

Fat 5g

Protein 15g

Carbohydrates 23g

Ingredients

1. 2 tsp. celery seed
2. 150 g of thick blue cheese dressing
3. 2-3 of low-fat buttermilk
4. 1/2 large red cabbage
5. 1/2 large green cabbage
6. 11/2 cup of green onion
7. Fresh-ground black pepper and salt to taste
8. 1/4-1/3 cup of crumbled blue cheese

Instructions

1. Mix the buttermilk and blue cheese dressing until it is thick enough.
2. Thickly slice the green onions. Use the Mandoline Slicer.
3. Mix the green cabbage, red cabbage, and the green onion in a bowl and add dressing.
4. Add the salt, celery seed, and fresh ground pepper and gently stir. Serve immediately.

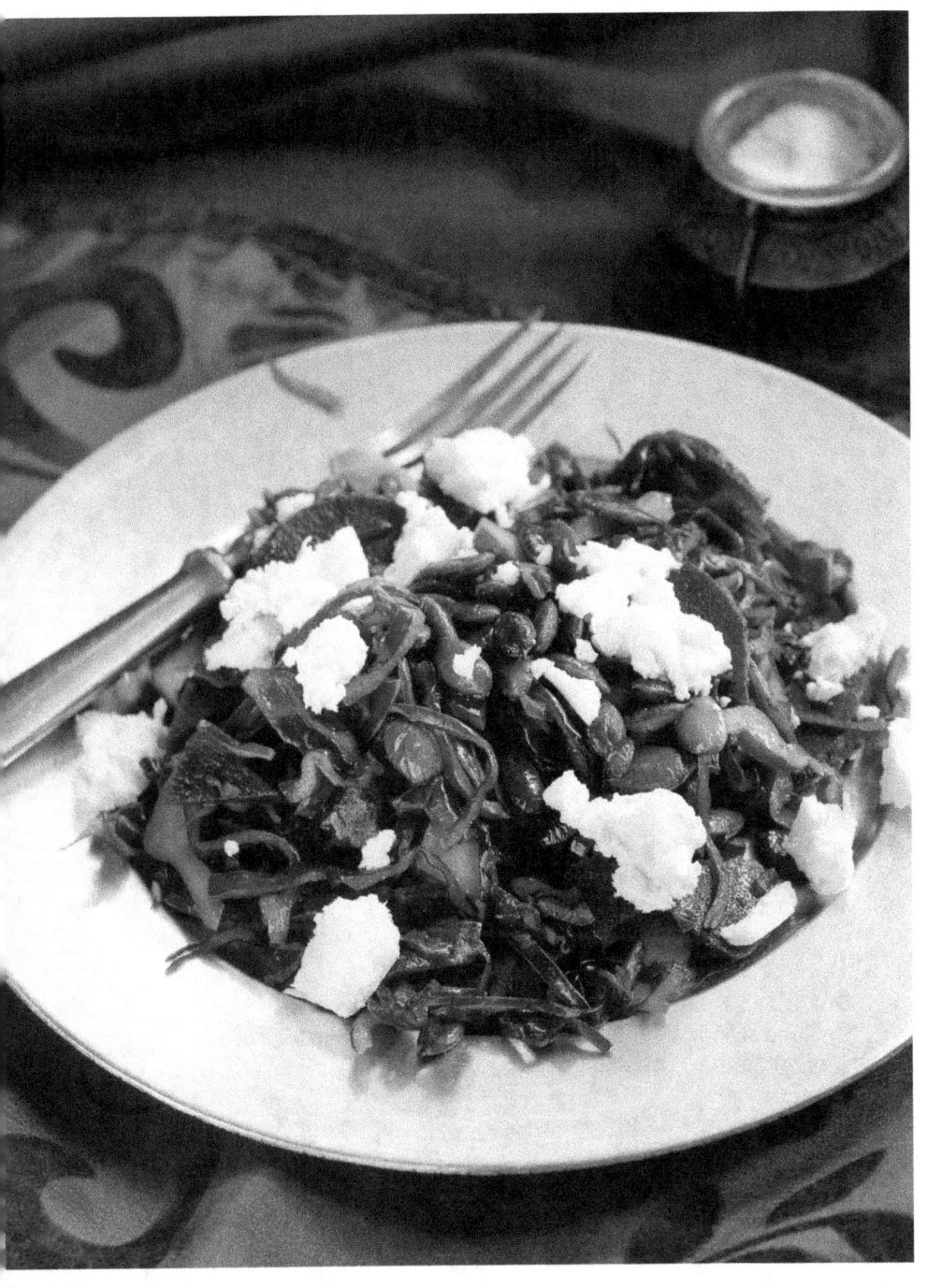

2. Steak Salad with Spicy Avocado Dressing

Preparation time 5 minutes

Calories 644

Carbohydrates 6g

Fat 53g

Protein 36g

Ingredients

Salad:

1. 2 grape tomatoes
2. 200 g rib eye cooked
3. salad greens
4. 1 cucumber
5. 1 avocado optional

Dressing:

1. 1 avocado
2. 1 cup fresh cilantro
3. 2 tablespoons lime juice
4. 2 tablespoons olive oil
5. 2 tablespoons red wine vinegar or balsamic vinegar
6. 1 clove garlic
7. 1/2 teaspoon sea salt

Instructions

1. Divide the salad ingredients into 2 separate plates.
2. In blender, mix all dressing ingredients. put it into 2 sm bowls, and serve with each salad.

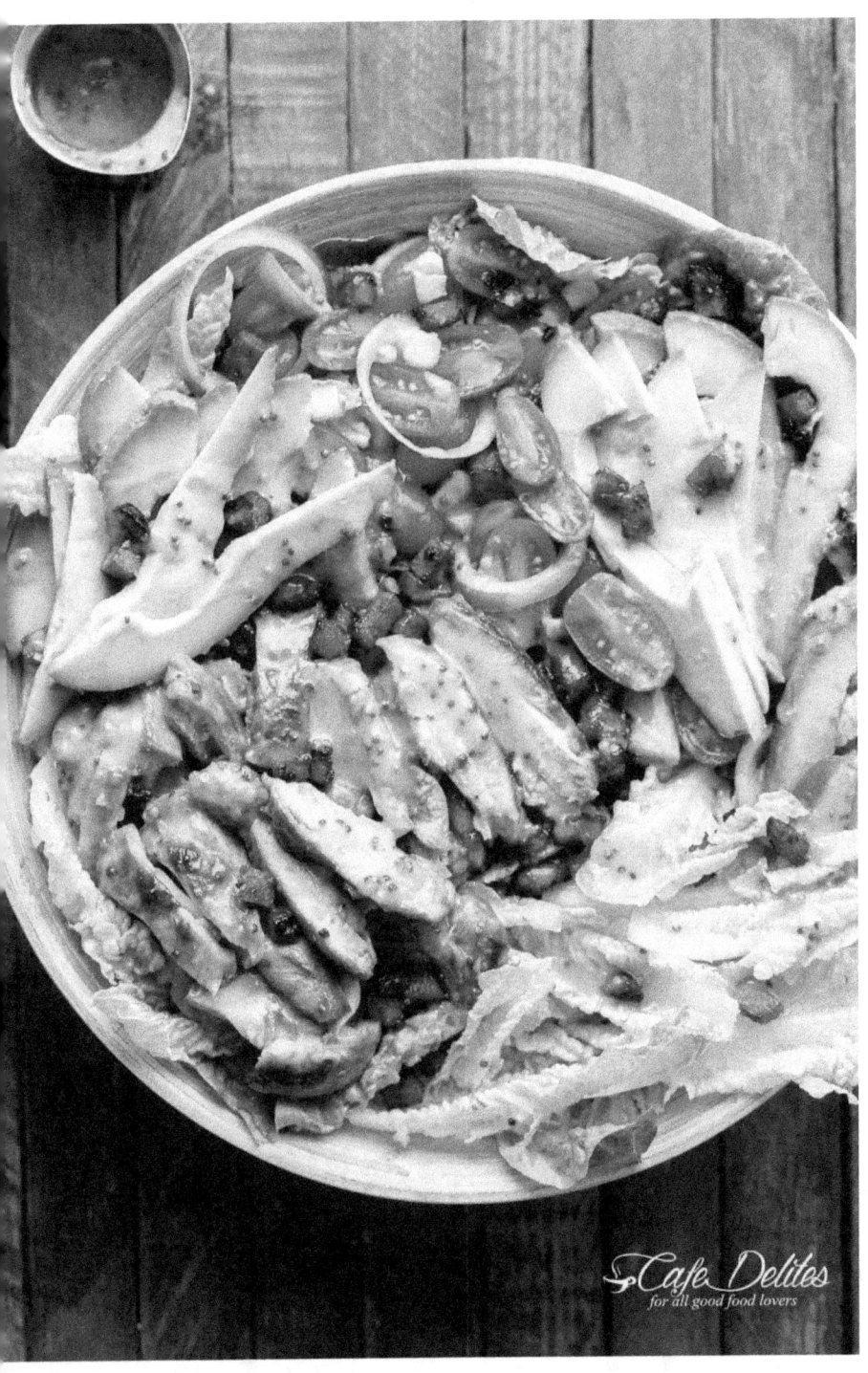

3. Oven-roasted Brussels sprouts with parmesan cheese

Preparation time 10 minutes

Calories 236

Carbohydrates 8 g

Fat 16 g

Protein 13 g

Ingredients

1. 3 tablespoons olive oil
2. 1⅓ lbs. of Brussels sprouts
3. 1 teaspoon dried thyme
4. 50 g parmesan cheese
5. Salt and pepper

Instructions

1. Preheat oven to 450°F
2. Trim your Brussels sprouts. Split in half.
3. Set in a baking dish. Pour olive oil on the top. Add thyme and pepper with salt.
4. Roast in oven for about 15–20 minutes. Shave parmesan cheese.
5. Serve

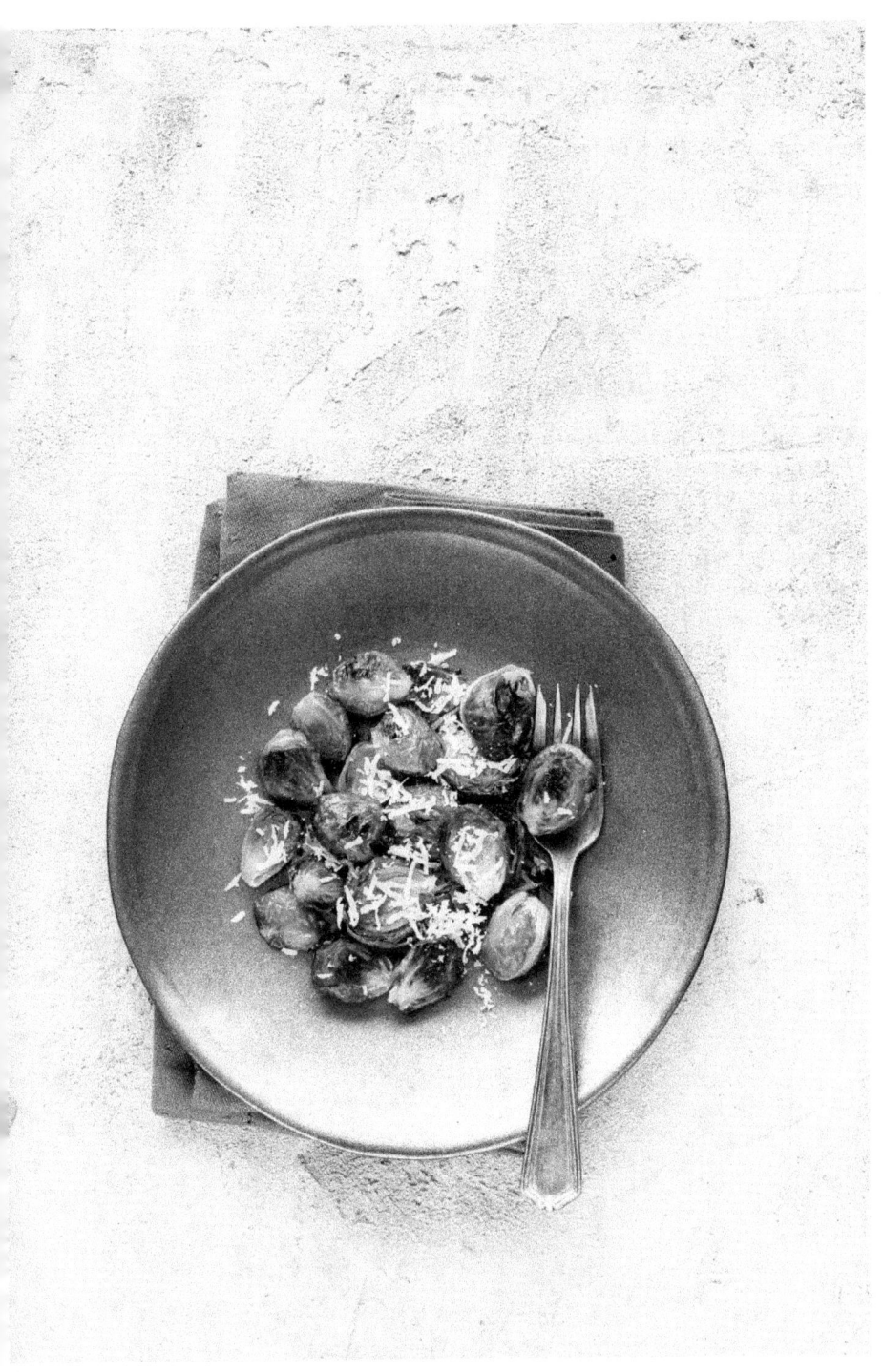

4. Arugula_Strawberry_Salad

Preparation time 10 minutes

Calories 228 kcal

Fat 21g

Protein 4g

Carbohydrates 7g

Ingredients

1. 6 organic strawberries quartered
2. 4 cups baby arugula
3. 1/4 cup sliced almonds
4. 2 tablespoons of Meyer lemon juice
5. Sea salt to taste
6. Meyer Lemon Vinaigrette
7. 2 tablespoons of avocado oil
8. Freshly ground pepper

Instructions

1. Layer strawberries, arugula, and almonds on plate.
2. For the Meyer Lemon Vinaigrette, mix Meyer lemon juice, salt, avocado oil and pepper.
3. Sprinkle vinaigrette over the salad and serve dressing on the side. Add additional fresh ground pepper and salt to taste.

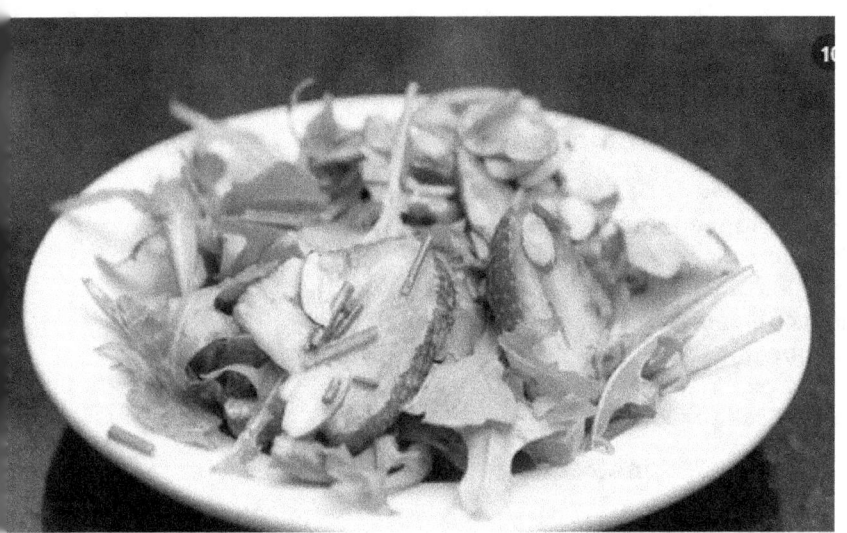

5. Kale and blueberry salad recipe

Preparation time: 5 minutes

Calories: 191

Fat: 16 g

Carbohydrates: 13 g

Protein: 4 g

Ingredients

1. 10 blueberries
2. 200 g kale, chopped roughly
3. 1 Tablespoon sliced almonds
4. 1/4 red onion, sliced thinly
5. 1 Tablespoon parsley
6. 1 Tsp lemon juice
7. 2 Tsp olive oil
8. Pepper and salt to taste

Instructions

1. Toss ingredients in a bowl together.
2. Serve in 2 plates

6. Green Salad with Italian Vinaigrette

reparation time: 10 minutes

alories 200

at 15g

arbohydrate 9g

rotein 5g

Ingredients for Salad:

1. 1 bunch radishes
2. 12-16 cups of salad greens
3. 1/4 medium red onion
4. 1 cucumber, sliced
5. 1 tomato

Ingredients for Italian Dressing:

1. ¼ cup apple cider vinegar
2. 6 tablespoons of extra-virgin olive oil
3. ¼ teaspoon of dried oregano leaves
4. ¼ teaspoon of dried marjoram leaves
5. ¼ teaspoon dried rosemary
6. ¼ teaspoon of dried thyme leaves
7. 1 clove garlic
8. 1/8 teaspoon of cracked pepper

Instructions

1. Combine salad ingredients in large salad bowl and mix well.
2. Blend the dressing ingredients in blender and puree.
3. Mix the entire salad and dressing before serving.

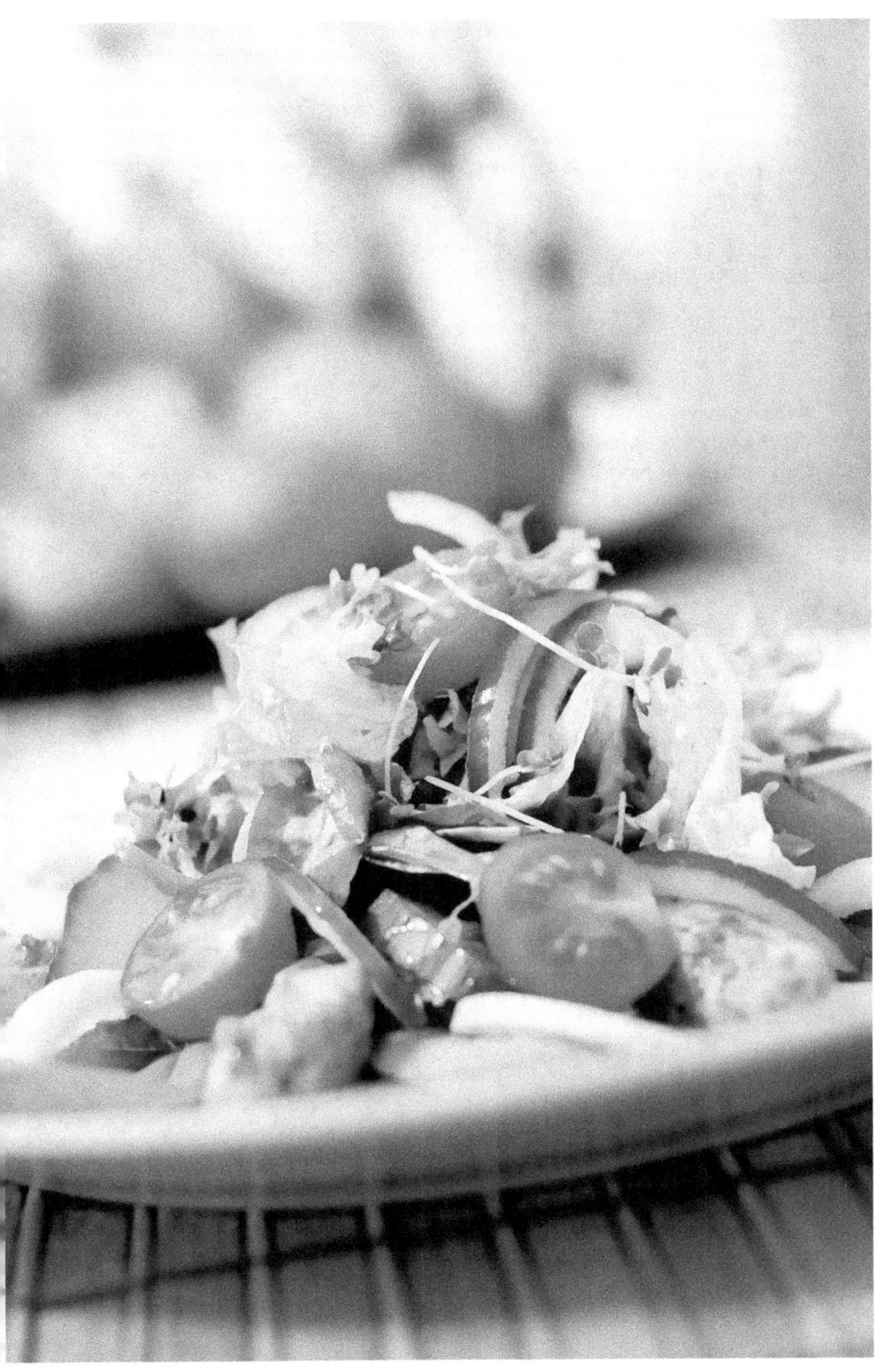

7. Arugula, Asparagus and Avocado

Breakfast Salad

Preparation time 5 minutes

Cook time 20 minutes

Ingredients

1. 1 tbsp olive oil
2. 20-25 stalks asparagus
3. Salt and pepper
4. 2 cups arugula
5. ½ avocado
6. 1 cup microgreens
7. 2 tbsp sunflower seeds
8. 2 eggs

Lemon Vinaigrette

1. 3 tsp lemon juice
2. 2 tbsp. olive oil
3. ¼ tsp Dijon mustard
4. ½ tsp, shallot
5. Salt and pepper

Instructions

1. Wash and slice the asparagus.
2. Olive oil in small pan lightly. Add the asparagus and season with pepper and salt and cook for two minutes.
3. Heat some water. Add the eggs and set timer for 6½ minutes. This is for soft-boiled eggs.
4. As the eggs boil, build an ice-water bath inside a bowl.
5. Make lemon vinaigrette by mixing all dressing ingredients together in a small bowl, set aside.
6. When eggs boil, remove them and submerge in your ice-water bath.
7. Assemble the salad by dividing the microgreens and arugula between two bowls. Then add the sunflower seeds and asparagus. Add a ¼ avocado
8. during each serving. Peel eggs, slice and add to the salads. Sprinkle lemon vinaigrette on top.

8. Chopped salad

Preparation time 10 minutes

Calories: 89

Fat 6.2g

Carb 7

Protein 4g

Ingredients

1. 1/2 tbsp. hemp seeds
2. ¾ lbs. spinach
3. 1 medium-size ripe tomato
4. 1/2 tbsp. hemp seeds
5. 1 tbsp. fried shallots
6. 1/2 tbsp. sunflower seeds

Dressing:

1. 1 ½ tsp of Red Boat fish sauce
2. ½ tsp sea salt
3. 1 tbsp. of fried shallot oil
4. Pinch of cayenne powder
5. Juice of 1 lime

Instructions

or shallot oil and fried shallots:

1. Slice one shallot thinly.
2. Heat your sauté pan with the coconut oil. Add sliced shallots.
3. Put the small pinch of salt. Stir shallots with your wooden spoon until it is golden brown.
4. Separate oil and crispy fried shallots. Set it aside for later.

or the salad:

1. Mix all the dressing ingredients.
2. Mix everything together with the shallot oil as well as fried shallots.

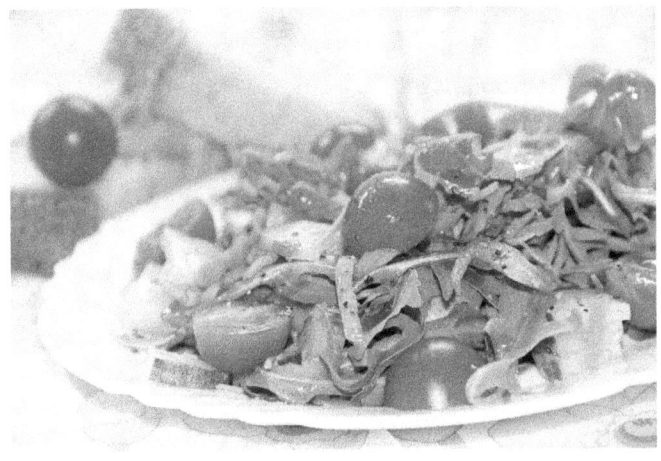

9. Tamari Marinated Steak Salad

Preparation time: 10 minutes

Calories 500

Carbohydrates 4 g

Fat 37g

Protein 33 g

Ingredients

1. 1/2 red bell pepper
2. 2 large handfuls of salad greens
3. 6-8 cherry tomatoes halved
4. 4 radishes, sliced
5. 1/2 Tablespoon of fresh lemon juice
6. 1 Tablespoon olive oil
7. 1/2 lb. steak
8. Salt to taste
9. Avocado oil for the steak
10. 1/4 cup of tamari soy sauce

Instructions

1. Marinade steak in tamari soy sauce.
2. Make the salad by mixing the tomatoes, bell pepper, adishes , as well as salad greens and lemon juice, olive oil, and salt.
3. Divide salad into 2 plates.
4. Put avocado oil in a frying pan and cook marinated steak.
5. Place steak on plate for a while. Cut steak into thin slices, and place slices on each salad.

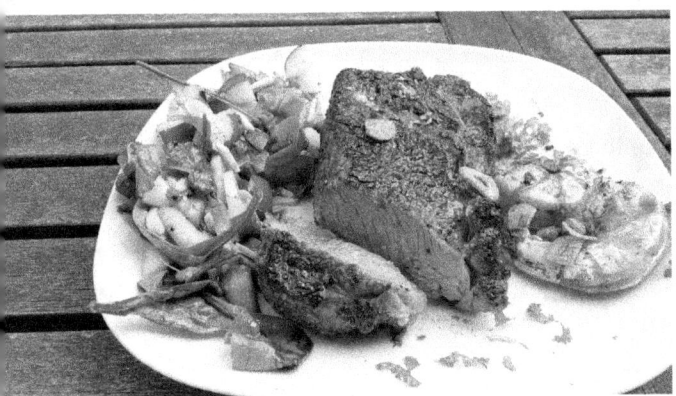

10. Smoked salmon salad

Preparation time: 5 minutes

Calories 650

Carbohydrates 10g

Protein 6g

Fat 42g

Ingredients

1. 1/2 cup blueberries
2. 8 oz smoked salmon
3. 2 Tablespoons olive oil
4. 100-150g salad greens
5. 1 Tablespoon of balsamic vinegar

Instructions

1. Mix salad greens and blueberries with the balsamic vinegar and olive oil.
2. Divide salad onto two plates. Top each plate with the smoked salmon halves.

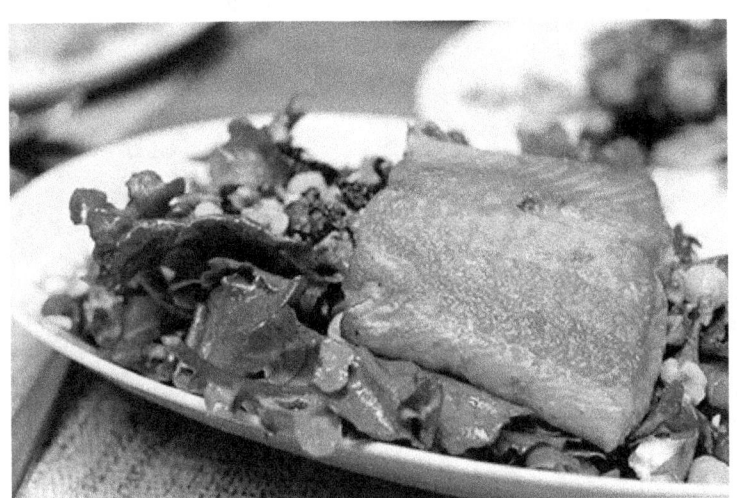

11. Quail egg salad

Preparation time: 10 minutes

Calories 195

Carbohydrates 31g

Protein 7.2 g

Fat 4.7 g

Ingredients

1. 15-20 grape tomatoes
2. 15 quail eggs
3. 1 head butter lettuce
4. 1 carrot, grated
5. Balsamic vinegar and olive oil
6. 50 g slices crispy bacon, crumbled
7. Salt to taste

Instructions

1. Put quail eggs in a boiling water for about 3 minutes for soft-boiled eggs. Leave longer for hard-boiled eggs.
2. Place eggs under running cold water to cool properly.
3. Peel eggs and rinse them.
4. Place the lettuce, tomatoes, bacon, and carrots into a salad bowl and add the balsamic vinegar, olive oil, and salt.
5. Add quail eggs to bowl and toss gently.

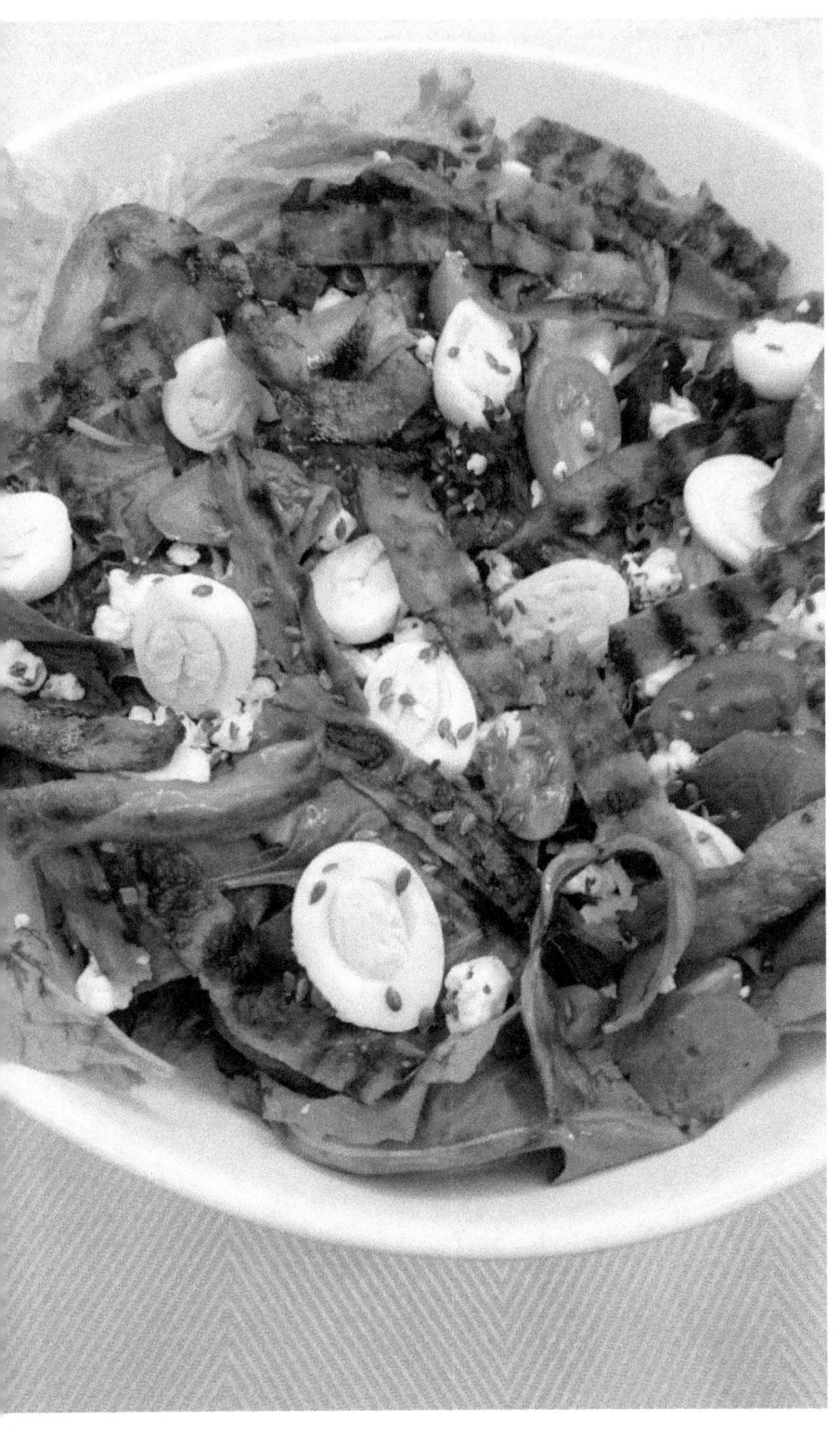

12. Kale Caesar Salad

Preparation time 20 minutes

Calories 640

Fat 51g

Sugar 5 g

Carbohydrates: 7 g

Protein 38 g

Ingredients

Salad:

1. 1 chicken breast
2. 2 slices bacon, diced
3. 1-Tablespoon coconut oil for cooking.
4. 2 eggs, hard-boiled or soft
5. 8 raspberries
6. Black pepper to taste
7. Baby kale leaves 125 g

Caesar salad dressing:

1. 1 anchovies
2. 1/4 cup Paleo Mayo
3. 1 cloves of garlic
4. 1/2 teaspoons mustard
5. Salt and pepper

Instructions

For salad dressing:

1. Blend salad dressing ingredients together.

For salad:

1. Put the coconut oil in a pan. Cook chicken breast and diced bacon.
2. Slice boiled eggs in half.
3. Add the salad dressing with kale leaves and top with the bacon, chicken, raspberries, and the egg halves.
Add extra black pepper to taste.

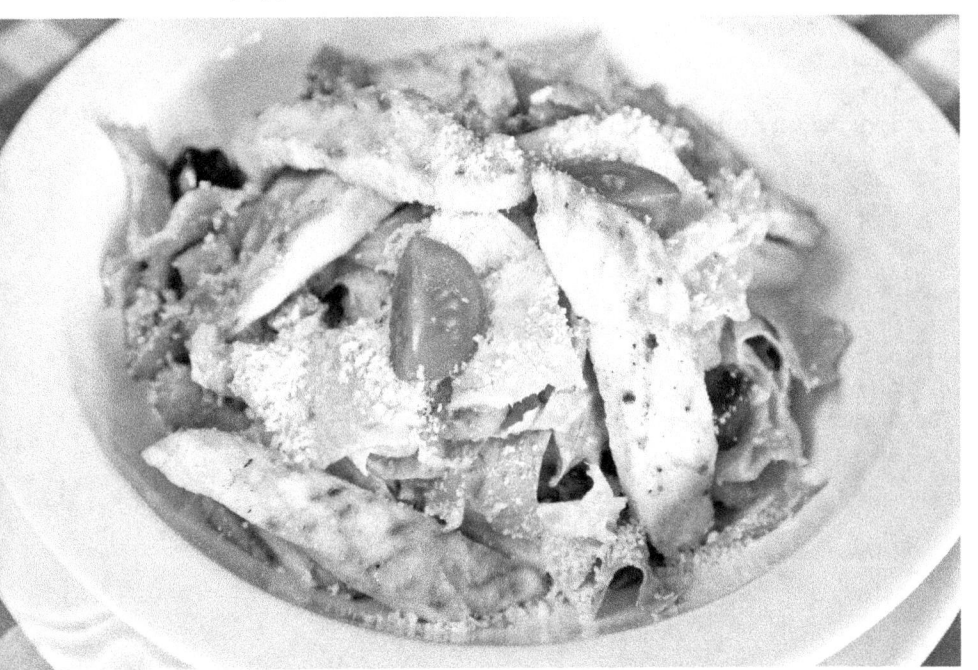

13. Sardine Salad

Preparation time: 5 minutes

Calories 400

Fat 34g

Carbohydrates 2g

Protein 30g

Ingredients

1. 120 g salad greens
2. 1 can sardine in brine or olive oil
3. 1 tomato
4. 1 egg
5. 60g bacon or deli meat or leftover meat
6. 1 tsp olive oil
7. 1 tsp lemon juice
8. Salt

Instructions

1. Prepare salad greens by mixing them with the lemon juice and olive oil.
2. Add deli meat in and mix.
3. Add tomato and egg.
4. Add salt to taste.

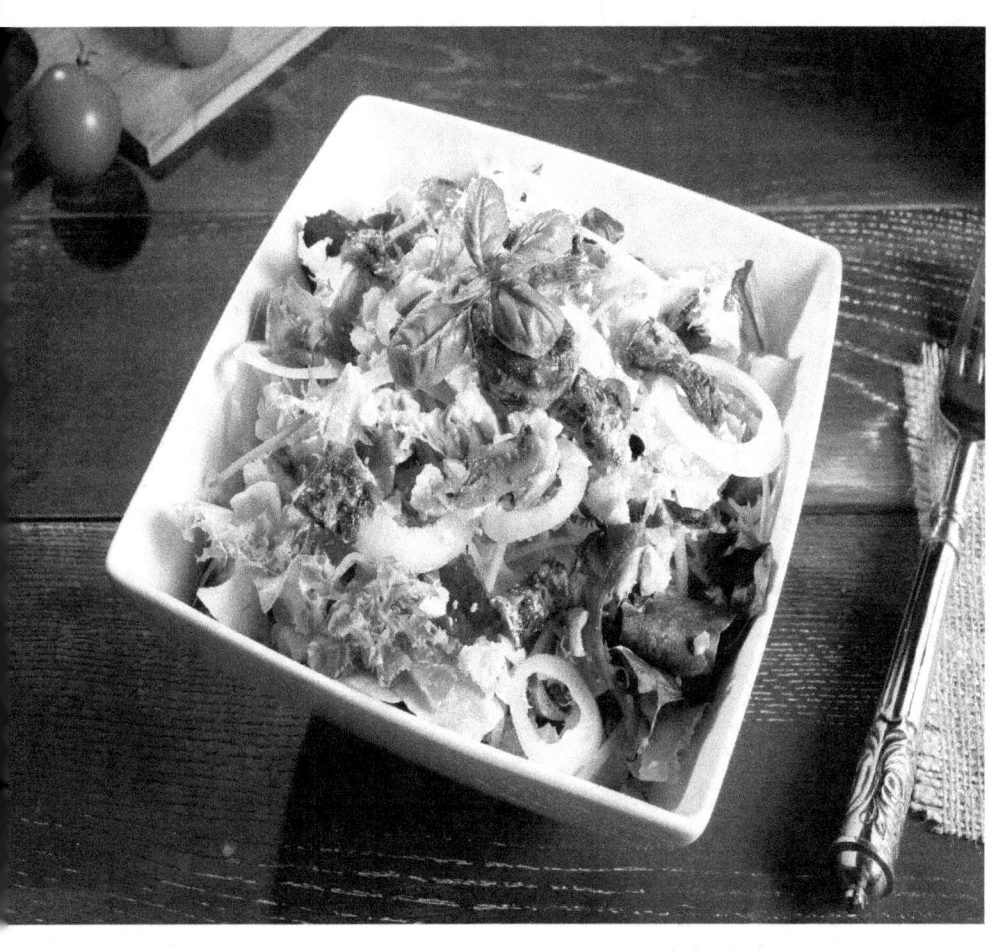

14. LCHF Caesar Salad

Preparation time 5 minutes

Calories 154

Fat 6.2

Carbohydrates 4g

Protein 12g

Ingredients

1. Sliced spring onions
2. Large handful leafy greens or baby kale
3. Cucumber cubes
4. 4 small tomatoes cut in half
5. Chicken
6. Parmesan
7. Blue cheese
8. Anchovies
9. Homemade mayonnaise

Instructions

1. Place the salad ingredients and the leafy greens at the bottom of a serving dish.
2. Put the cheeses and chicken on top.
3. Add the anchovies to finish it off.
4. Sprinkle homemade mayonnaise.

15. Chicken Shawarma Salad

Preparation Time 10 minutes

Calories 746

Fat 56 g

Protein 50 g

Carbohydrates 11 g

Ingredients

Salad dressing:

1. 1 Tablespoon lemon juice
2. 3 Tablespoons olive oil
3. Salt and black pepper

Chicken pieces:

1. 1 tsp cumin powder
2. 2 chicken breasts cubed
3. 1 tsp paprika
4. 1 tsp onion powder
5. 1 tsp garlic powder
6. 1 tsp Italian seasoning
7. Pinch of cayenne pepper
8. 4 Tablespoons avocado oil
9. Salt to taste

Salad:

1. 1/2 cucumber, sliced
2. 1 head of romaine lettuce
3. 1/4 red onion
4. Handful fresh parsley

Instructions

For dressing:

1. Whisk dressing ingredients in a small bowl.
2. Using another bowl, add all dry ingredients for chicken.
3. Place chicken pieces in the bowl and cover with spices.
4. In a pan, heat the avocado oil. Cook chicken until tender.

For salad:

1. Toss salad ingredients with salad dressing and put cooked chicken pieces on the top.

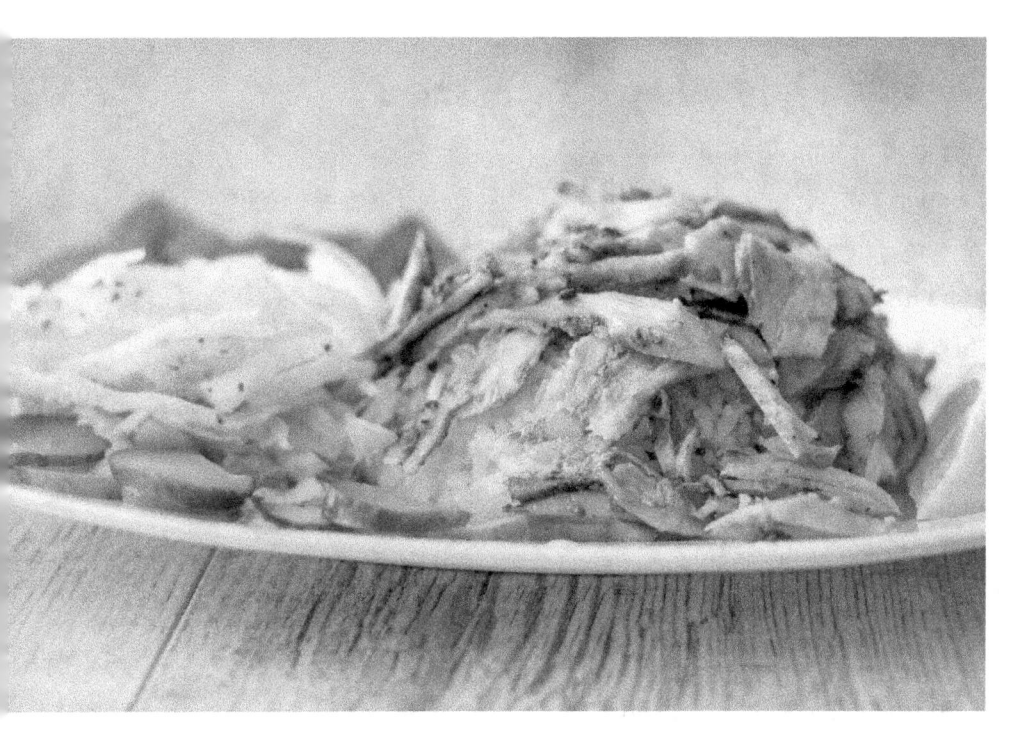

16. Simple Taco Salad

Preparation time 10 minutes

Calories 332

Carbohydrates 2g

Protein 7g

Fat 6.5g

Ingredients

1. 1 large onion
2. 450 g of ground beef
3. taco spice
4. 2 Roma tomatoes
5. Homemade guacamole
6. 4 handfuls fresh spinach leaves
7. 2 jalapeños papers , sliced
8. 4 tsp slivered almonds
9. 1/2 cup of diced nopalitos
10. Chopped cilantro leaves

Instructions

1. In cast iron skillet, heat the onion, ground beef, taco spice and two tablespoons of water.
2. Mix guacamole ingredients.
Divide ingredients into four separate plates.

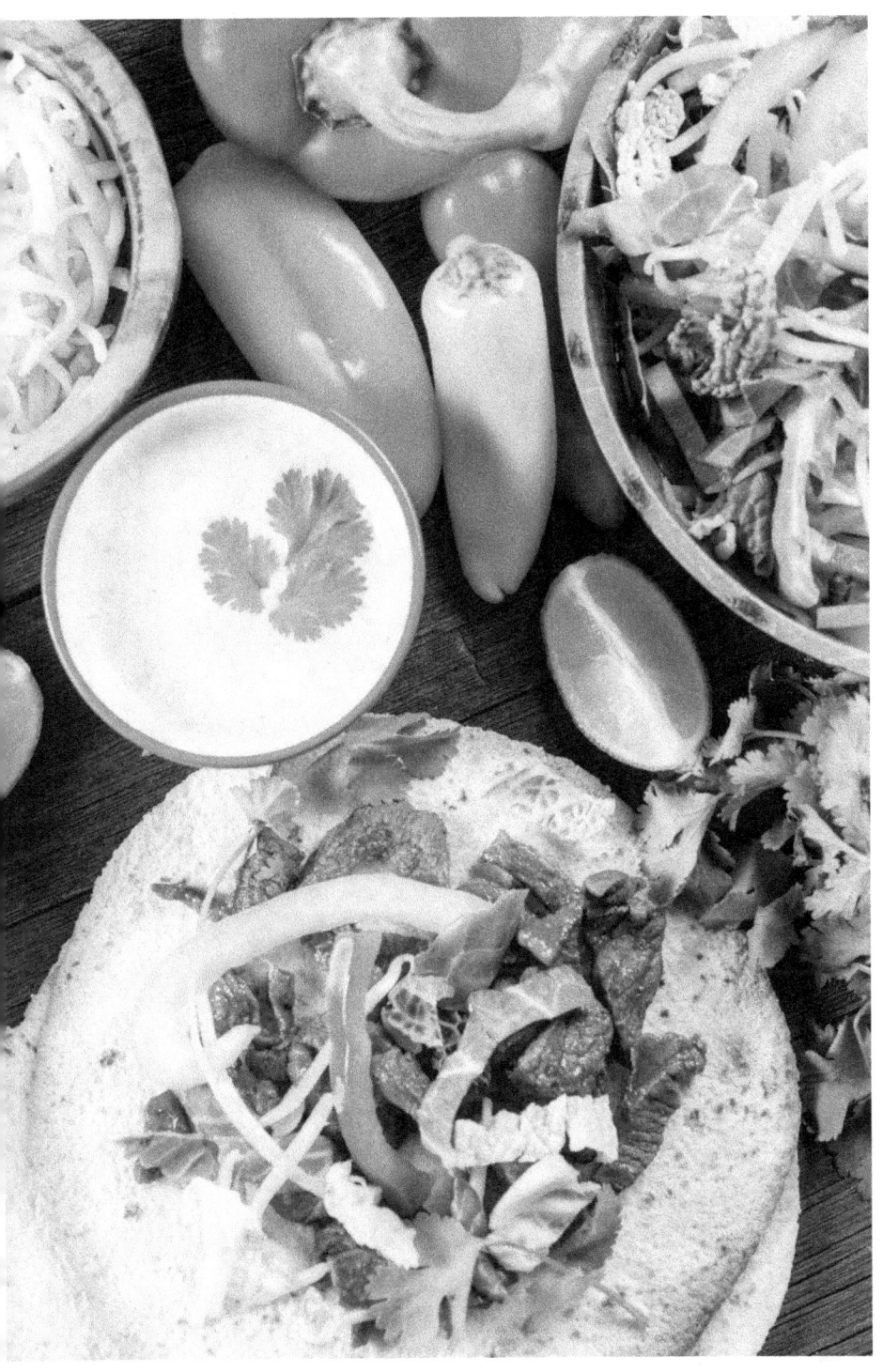

17. Cobb Salad

Preparation Time 10 minutes

Calories 518

Fat 43g

Protein 20g

Carbohydrates 12g

Ingredients

1. 7 cherry tomatoes
2. 2 heads romaine lettuce
3. 1 avocado
4. 5 slices of pastured bacon
5. 3 pastured eggs

Chicken dressing

1. 1 tbsp of olive oil
2. 1 boneless skinless pastured chicken breast
3. 1/2 tsp sea salt
4. 1/2 tsp of garlic powder
5. 1/2 tsp black pepper
6. 1/2 tsp of paprika

Dressing:

1. 2 tbsp balsamic vinegar
2. 2 tbsp of olive oil
3. 1/2 tsp black pepper
4. 1/2 tsp sea salt

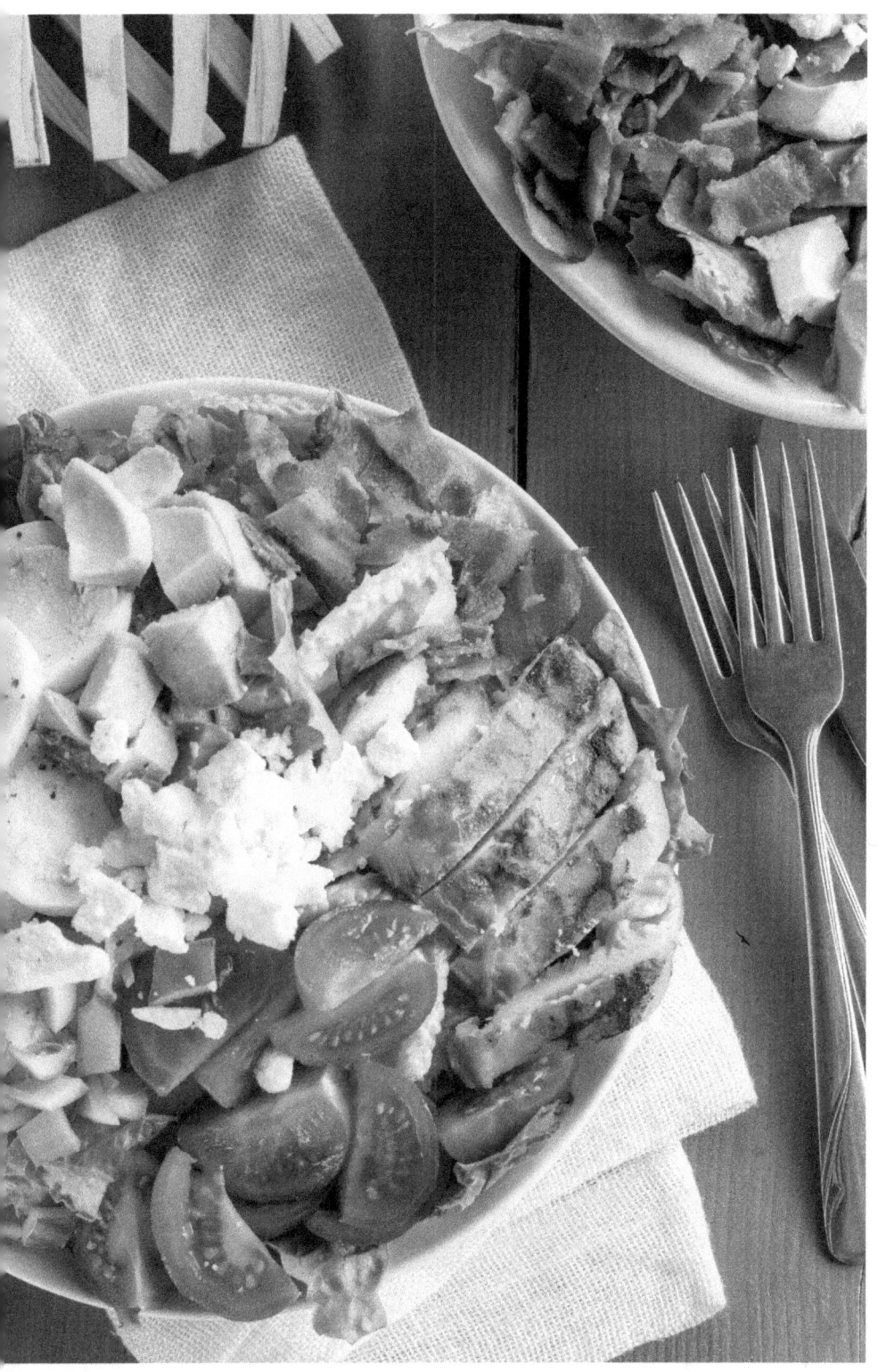

Instructions

Salad dressing:

1. Blend all the dressing ingredients in a jar and cover
using an airtight lid. Then shake thoroughly until all ingredients mix.

Chicken breast

1. Brine the chicken. Fill bowl with hand-hot water and add
1 tsp sea salt. Put chicken in a salt-water bowl for 15 minutes.
2. Pre-heat oven to 425°.
3. Remove chicken and pat dry with paper towel. Set in pyres
baking dish. Brush with olive oil. Add garlic powder, salt, pepper,
and paprika and rub it in.
4. Put in oven and bake for 15-20 minutes. Remove the chicken
from oven and allow it rest for 15 minutes before cutting.

Bacon:

1. Place strips in a cast iron pan, and turn heat to low medium.
Let the bacon cook, flip every few minutes.
2. Remove it and set on a paper towel.
3. When the bacon cools, transfer it to the cutting board.
Chop it into tiny bits.

Hard-boiled eggs:

1. Place eggs in pot and fill it to cover them with cold water.
2. Pour a dash of vinegar and a dash of salt. Increase heat and let the water come to a boil. When it does, turn off heat and remove pot from burner.
3. Cover pot and let it sit for 10-15 minutes.
4. Drain hot water from pan and rinse the eggs with cold water. When the eggs have cooled, peel, then chop and set aside.

Salad:

1. Wash and chop romaine lettuce and pat dry.
2. Place lettuce in a bowl. Cut the chicken, avocado, and tomatoes into tiny pieces. Arrange the chopped toppings into small rows over romaine lettuce.
Sprinkle the dressing over salad and serve!

18. Summer Berry Salad

Preparation time 15 minutes

Calories 432

Protein 13g

Carbohydrates 12g

Fat 5.6g

Ingredients

1. 1 Chicken Breast
2. 1 head Romaine Lettuce
3. Paleo Adobo Seasoning
4. ½ cup Blueberries
5. 5-6 Strawberries
6. ¼ cup Toasted Almonds
7. Lemon basil salad dressing

Instructions

1. Dust chicken lightly with Paleo Adobo Seasoning.
Bake, grill, or pan-fry and cut the chicken after allowing
it to rest.

2. Chop lettuce and blend with sliced strawberries, slice
grilled chicken, blueberries, lemon basil salad dressing and
toasted almonds.

19. Calamari Salad

Preparation time 10 minutes

Calories 432

Protein 16g

Carbohydrates 6g

Fat 12g

Ingredients

1. 1 tsp coconut oil
2. 450-500 g calamari
3. 1/2 tsp sea salt
4. 1/4 cup of red wine vinegar
5. 1 small onion
6. 3 garlic cloves
7. 1 1/2 limes
8. 15 small tomatoes
9. bed of greens
10. Extra-virgin olive oil
11. Ground pepper

Instructions

1. On medium heat in a skillet, heat sea salt, coconut oil, calamari, onion, vinegar, garlic cloves and juice of 1 lime. Cook for 5 minutes until onions are tender or the calamari are dense.
2. Drain skillet ingredients.
3. Divide the greens into 3 to 4 plates. Scoop the calamari mixture on each bed of greens and add tomato halves.
4. Sprinkle with juice of lime and olive oil. Sprinkle with the ground pepper.

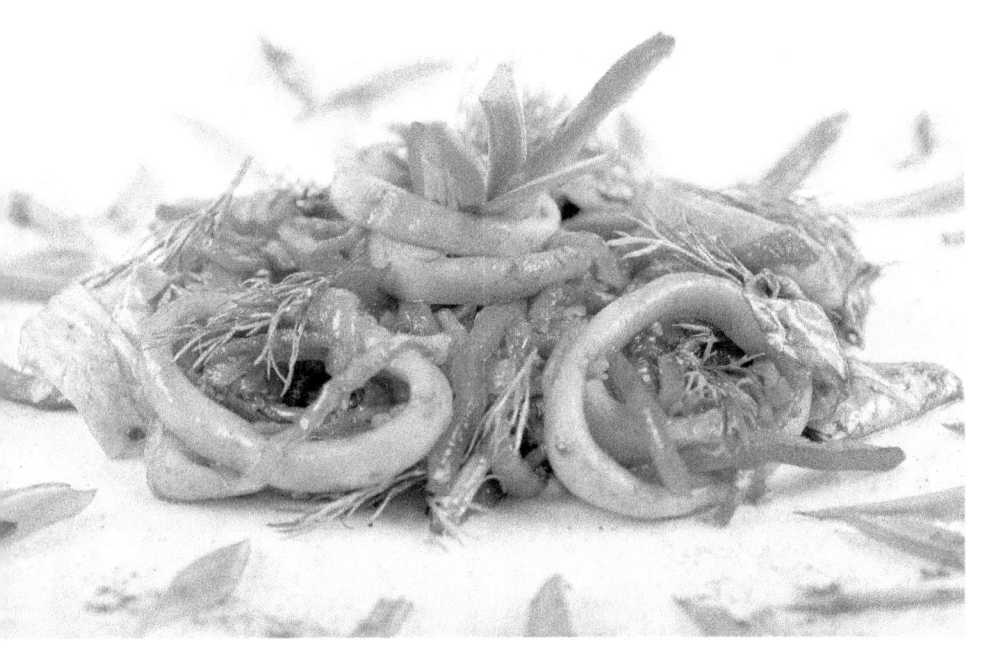

20. Shrimp and arugula salad

Preparation time 5 minutes

Calories 264

Protein 6g

Carbohydrates 3g

Fat 13g

Instructions

1. 450 g large shrimp, cooke
2. baby arugula
3. 4 tbsp. olive oil
4. 1 avocado diced
5. Fresh cracked pepper
6. 2 lemons
7. Sea salt

Instructions

1. Add the avocado, arugula, and shrimp to a large bowl.
Sprinkle the juice of 1 lemon, half the olive oil quantity, and pepper
and salt to taste.
2. Mix lightly, and add more olive oil. Taste and adjust the
seasonings.
3. Serve with the lemon wedges on each side.

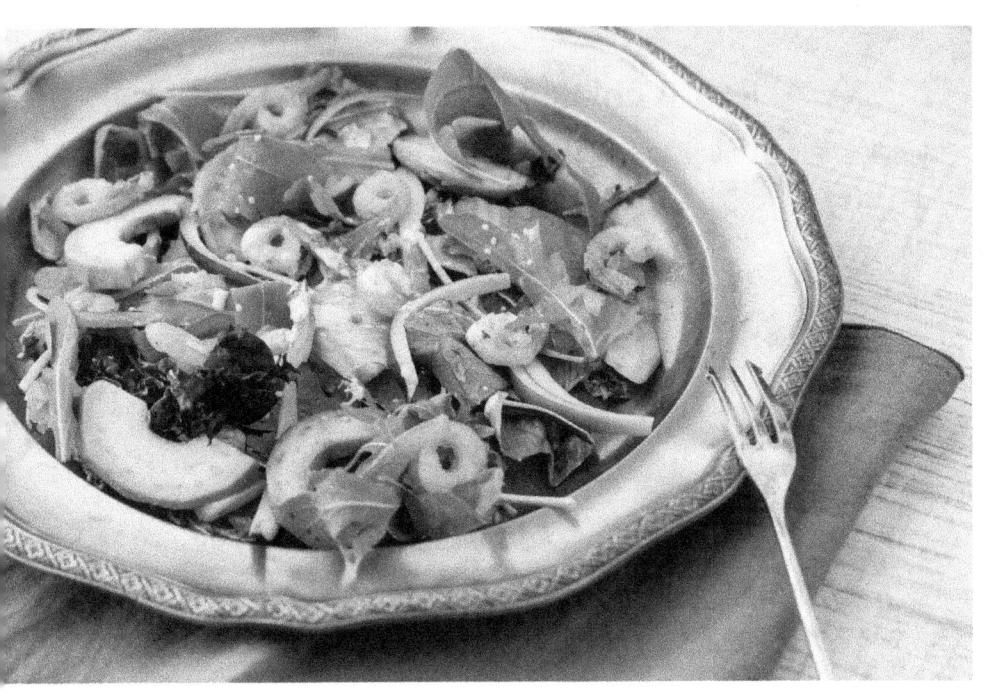

21. Pesto chicken avocado salad

Preparation time 10 minutes

Calories 212

Protein 9g

Carbohydrates 5g

Fat 14g

Ingredients

Dressing:

1. 1/2 tsp dried basil
2. 3/4 cup olive oil
3. 1/4 cup of balsamic vinegar
4. 1 clove of garlic
5. Pepper and salt

Pesto:

1. ½ clove of garlic
2. 1 large bunch of basil leaves
3. 1/3 cup olive oil
4. ¼ cup pine nuts
5. ¼ tsp unrefined sea salt

Salad:

1. 1 tbsp. butter
2. 4 boneless and skinless chicken thighs
3. 2 cloves garlic
4. 1/4 tsp salt
5. 1 avocado
6. 5 cups romaine lettuce
7. 1 cup cherry tomatoes
8. 1/4 cup pine nuts
9. Basil leaves

Instructions

Dressing:

1. Combine all the dressing ingredients in glass jar, place lid on, and then shake vigorously.

Pesto:

1. Place garlic and basil leaves into food processor.
Process until broken up into paste. Add salt and olive oil and keep processing until smooth.
2. Add hemp seed, pine nuts, pumpkin, macadamia nuts, and pulse until it reaches the desired consistency.

Chicken:

1. Sprinkle melted fat, salt and crushed garlic over the chicken thighs. Stir.
2. Preheat grill.
3. Put thighs on grill
4. Grill on each side until it is browned.
5. When it is cooked, remove from the grill and set in a bowl.
6. Sprinkle the 1/4 cup pesto, stir, and set aside.

Salad:

1. Place the lettuce in a large bowl.
2. Cut chicken into small strips and place on the top.
3. Add avocado, sliced tomatoes, and pine nuts.
4. Top with the basil strips.
5. Drizzle on the dressing.

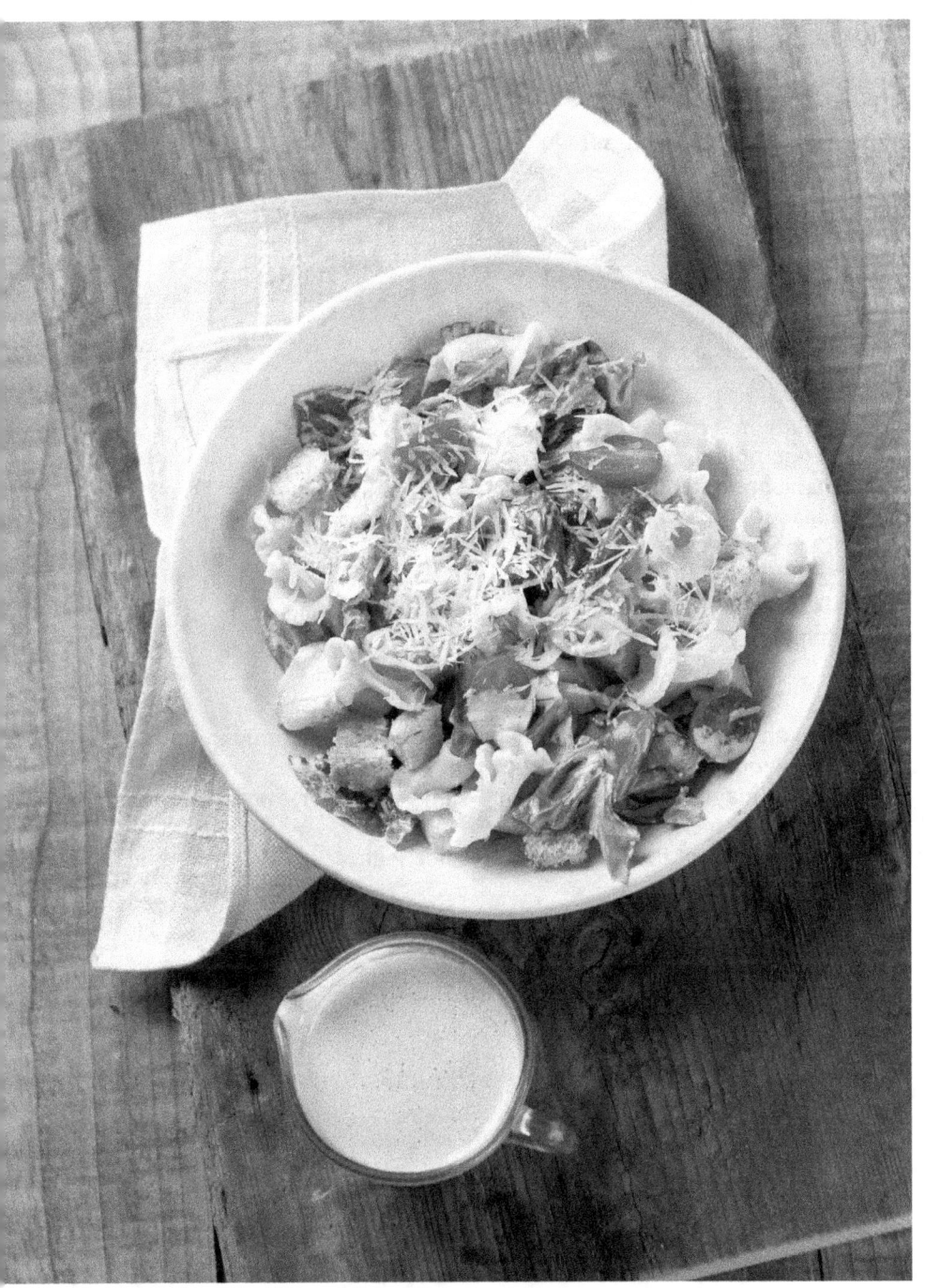

22. Avocado Egg Salad Wraps

Preparation Time 10 minutes

Calories 178 kcal

Fat 14g

Carbohydrates 6g

Protein 7g

Ingredients

1. 1 medium Avocado
2. 4 eggs boiled
3. 3 tablespoons mayonnaise
4. 2 teaspoons Lemon Juice
5. 1/2 teaspoons Salt
6. 2 tablespoons chives
7. 1/4 teaspoon Pepper
8. Romaine

Instructions

1. With an egg slicer, cut the boiled eggs and add to mixing bowl.
2. Dice avocado and add it to the eggs.
3. Put the mayonnaise, lemon juice, chives, pepper, and salt to the bowl and blend gently.
4. Add a ¼ cup of the mix into the lettuce leaf.

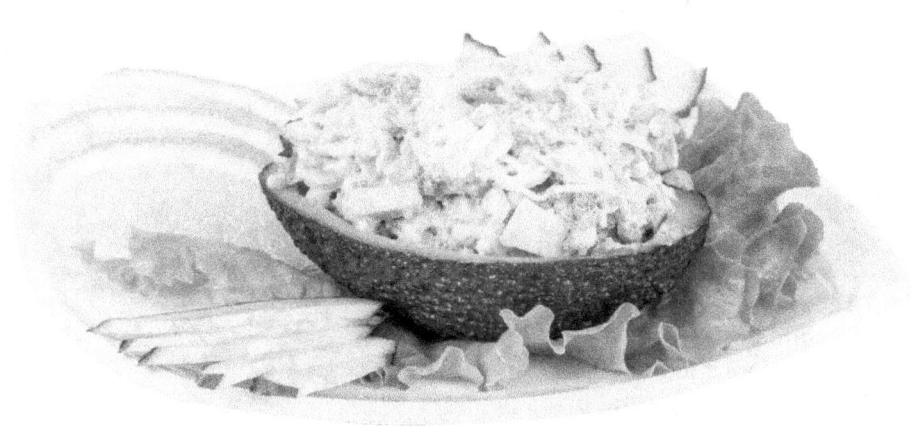

23. Creamy keto cucumber

Preparation Time: 5 minutes

Calories 116

Fat12 g

Carbohydrates 2 g

Protein 1 g

Ingredients

1. 2 Tablespoons of mayo
2. 1 cucumber
3. 2 Tablespoons lemon juice
4. Salt and freshly ground black pepper

Instruction

1. Mix the mayo, cucumber slices, and lemon juice together. Add pepper and salt to taste.

24. Seaweed (kombu) salad

Preparation Time: 10 minutes

Calories 202

Protein 6g

Carbohydrates 6.1g

Fat 9g

Ingredients

1. 4 cloves of garlic
2. 1 lb. fresh kombu seaweed
3. 2 tsp. apple cider vinegar
4. 2 tsp. coconut aminos
5. 2 Tablespoons sesame oil
6. 2 red peppers
7. Salt to taste

Instructions

1. Boil kombu in water for about 30 minutes, then cool before slicing into thin strips.
2. Mix well with the sesame oil, apple cider vinegar, crushed garlic, and coconut aminos
3. Add the salt to taste as well as chopped red peppers.

25. Avocado salad

Preparation Time: 5 minutes

Calories 432

Carbohydrate 4g

Protein 11g

Ingredients

1. 1 tsp olive oil
2. 75 g salad
3. 1 ripe avocado
4. 100 g bacon
5. 1 tsp balsamic vinegar
6. Salt

Instructions

1. Split the ripe avocado.
2. Remove its pit, and cut each half into small cubes.
Then scoop out the avocado with a spoon.
3. Add bacon and salad.
4. Toss with balsamic vinegar, extra virgin
 olive oil, and salt.

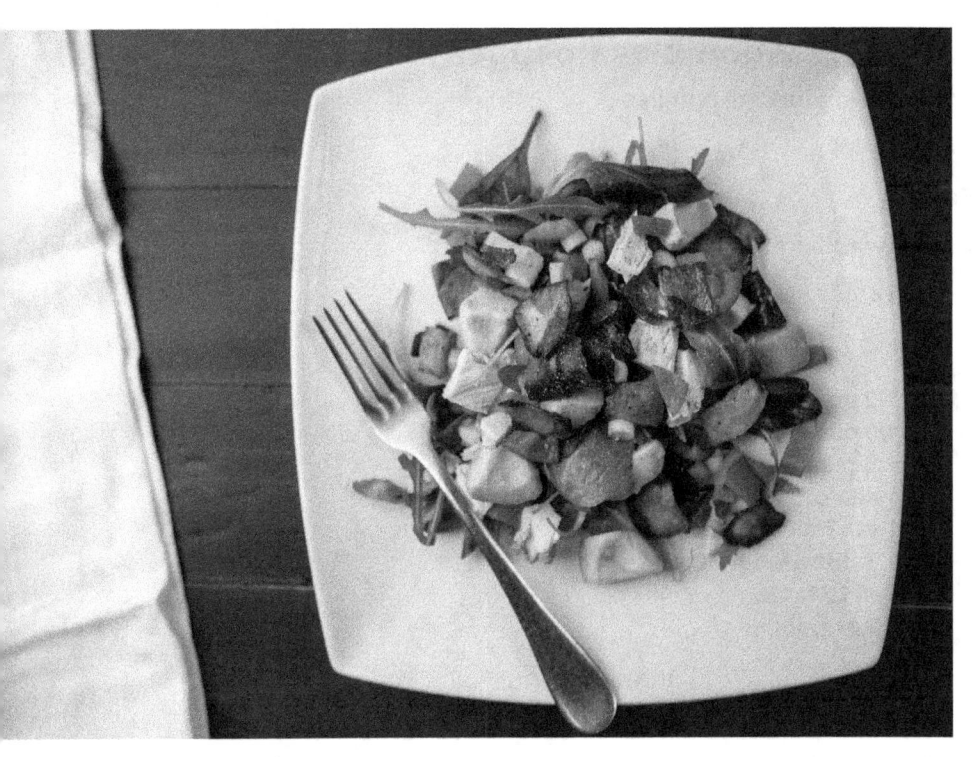

26. Lemon black pepper tuna salad

Preparation Time: 10 minutes

Calories 480

Fat 40 g

Carbohydrates 11 g

Protein 45 g

Ingredients

1. 1/2 small avocado
2. 1/3 cucumber
3. 1 tsp lemon juice
4. 1 can of tuna
5. 1 tsp Paleo mayo
6. 1 Tablespoon mustard
7. Salt to taste
8. Black pepper

Instructions

1. Mix the avocado and diced cucumber with lemon juice.
2. Flake tuna and mix properly with the mustard and mayo.
3. Add tuna to cucumber and avocado. Add salt.
4. Place tuna salad on salad greens.
5. Sprinkle the black pepper on the top.

27. TOMATO MOZZARELLA SALAD

Preparation time 10 minutes

Calories 245

Fat 23g

Carbohydrates 30g

Protein 16g

Ingredients

1. 2 logs of mozzarella cheese
2. 4-5 tomatoes
3. Fresh basil leaves
4. Fresh ground black pepper and sea salt
5. Extra-virgin olive oil
6. 2 cups of balsamic vinegar
7. Balsamic Reduction

Instructions

1. In a casserole dish, arrange mozzarella, slices of tomatoes, and basil vertically, until you create two rows.
2. Sprinkle olive oil on the top, followed by a dash of balsamic reduction.
3. Drizzle with fresh ground pepper and sea salt.

1. Using a small saucepan, boil the balsamic vinegar over medium-low heat.
2. Cool and keep covered in your refrigerator. Expose to room temperature prior to use.

28. CABBAGE AND CUCUMBER SALAD

Preparation time 10 minutes

Calories 206

Protein 12g

Carbohydrates 30g

Fat 6g

Ingredients

1. 2 Persian cucumbers
2. 1/2 head of white cabbage
3. 2 tablespoons of fresh dill
4. 2 tablespoons of green onions
5. 2 teaspoon of unrefined salt
6. 1/2 lemon, juiced
7. 3 tablespoons avocado oil
8. Salt and pepper

Instructions

1. Chop cabbage and season with a teaspoon of salt.
2. Mix with hands pressing into cabbage to release natural juices.
3. Add the green onions, chopped cucumbers, and fresh dill.
4. Squeeze one lemon and get the juice. Add salt and pepper.
 Pour the oil and mix well.

29. Easy Keto Broccoli Slaw

Preparation time 10 minutes

Calories 110

Fat 10g

Carbohydrates 2g

Protein 2g

Ingredient

1. 1 1/2 Tbsp. of apple cider vinegar
2. 1 Tbsp. of olive oil
3. 1 Tbsp. of Dijon mustard
4. 1/3 cup of sugar-free mayonnaise
5. 1 tsp celery seeds
6. 2 Tbsp. of granulated sugar substitute
7. 1/2 tsp kosher salt
8. 4 cups of bagged broccoli slaw
9. 1/4 tsp of black pepper

Instructions

1. Whisk the mayonnaise, olive oil, apple cider vinegar, celery seeds, mustard, sugar substitute, salt and pepper in a bowl until fully combined. Pour the broccoli slaw. Mix well to coat.

30. Avocado Tuna Salad

Preparation Time 10 minutes

Calories 216

Protein 3g

Carbohydrates 13g

Fat 4g

Ingredients

1. 1 English cucumber
2. 3 small cans of tuna in oil
3. 2 large avocados
4. 1 small red onion
5. 1/2 bunch of cilantro
6. 2 Tbsp. of lemon juice
7. 2 Tbsp. of olive oil
8. 1/8 tsp of black pepper
9. 1 tsp sea salt

Instructions

1. Combine the sliced avocado, sliced cucumber,
red onion, 1/4 cup cilantro and drained tuna in bowl.
2. Sprinkle salad ingredients with the lemon juice, olive
oil, salt and black pepper. Toss to combine.

31. Low Carb Pasta Salad

reparation time 15 minutes

alories 290

rotein 4g

arbohydrates 30

at 6g

Ingredients

1. 1/2 cup of Creamy Italian Dressing
2. 4 medium-sized zucchini
3. 1/2 cup of black olives
4. 1/4 cup of banana pepper rings
5. 1 oz pepperoni
6. 1 oz Genoa salami
7. 8 cherry tomatoes
8. Salt and pepper

Instructions

1. Make zucchini noodles
2. Combine banana peppers, zucchini black olives, pepperoni, and salami in a bowl.
3. Pour the Creamy Italian Dressing on top and mix to coat.
4. Refrigerate for an hour.
5. Before serving, add tomatoes and toss.

32. Zucchini salad

Preparation Time 20 minutes

Calories 246

Fat 10g

Carbohydrates 31g

Protein 8g

Ingredients

Peanut sauce:

1. 1/2 tbsp. of rice wine vinegar
2. 1 tbsp. water
3. 2 tbsp. of creamy natural peanut butter
4. 1/2 tbsp. of coconut sugar
5. 2 tsp tamari
6. 1/2 tbsp. of sriracha

Zucchini/cucumber noodle salad:

1. 1 large bell pepper
2. 2 medium zucchini
3. 2 medium cucumbers
4. 1 large peach
5. 1/4 medium white onion
6. Instant peanut sauce
7. Green onions
8. Sesame seeds

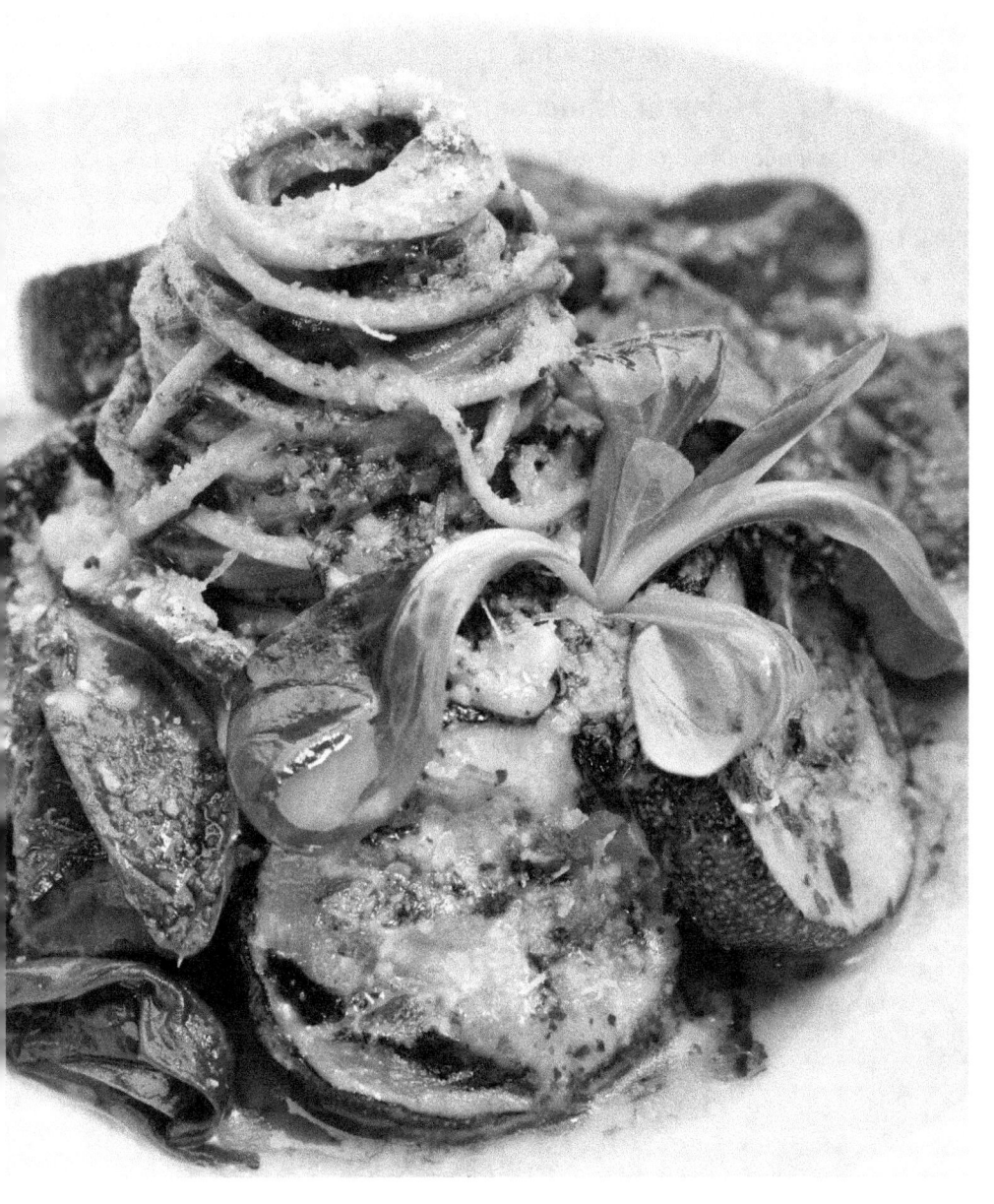

Instructions

Instant peanut sauce:

1. Mix the coconut sugar, peanut butter, rice wine vinegar sriracha. and tamari until a smooth paste is formed.

Salad:

1. Sprinkle cucumbers and spiralized zucchini generously with salt. Set in colander to drain the liquid.
2. Rinse off salt from noodles and pat dry using a towel. Gently mix with the onion, bell pepper, and peach.
3. Add the peanut sauce and serve immediately.

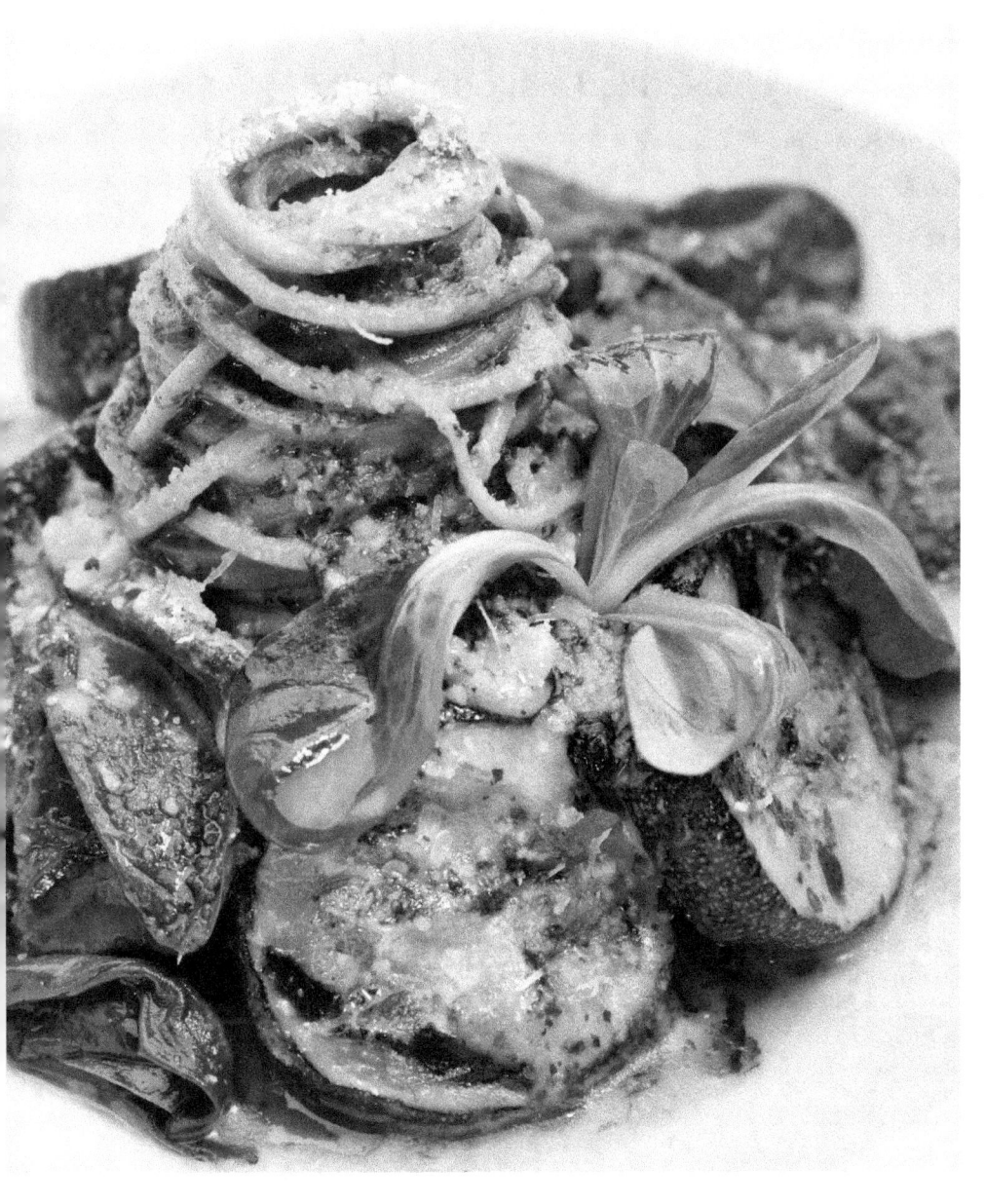

33. Grilled Halloumi Salad

Preparation time 10 minutes

560 Calories

Fat 47g

Protein 21g

Carbohydrates 7g

Ingredients

1. 1 Persian cucumber
2. 100 g halloumi cheese
3. 1 handful baby arugula
4. 5 grape tomatoes
5. 150 g chopped walnuts
6. Balsamic vinegar
7. Olive oil
8. Salt

Instructions

1. Cut your halloumi cheese into small slices but not too thin.
2. Grill the halloumi for 3-5 minutes side by side.
3. Start making the salad. Wash and cut your veggies and combine in the salad bowl.
4. Wash your baby arugula and add it as well.
5. When grill marks show on the halloumi, arrange it on your salad, drizzle some salt and then dress with balsamic vinegar and olive oil.

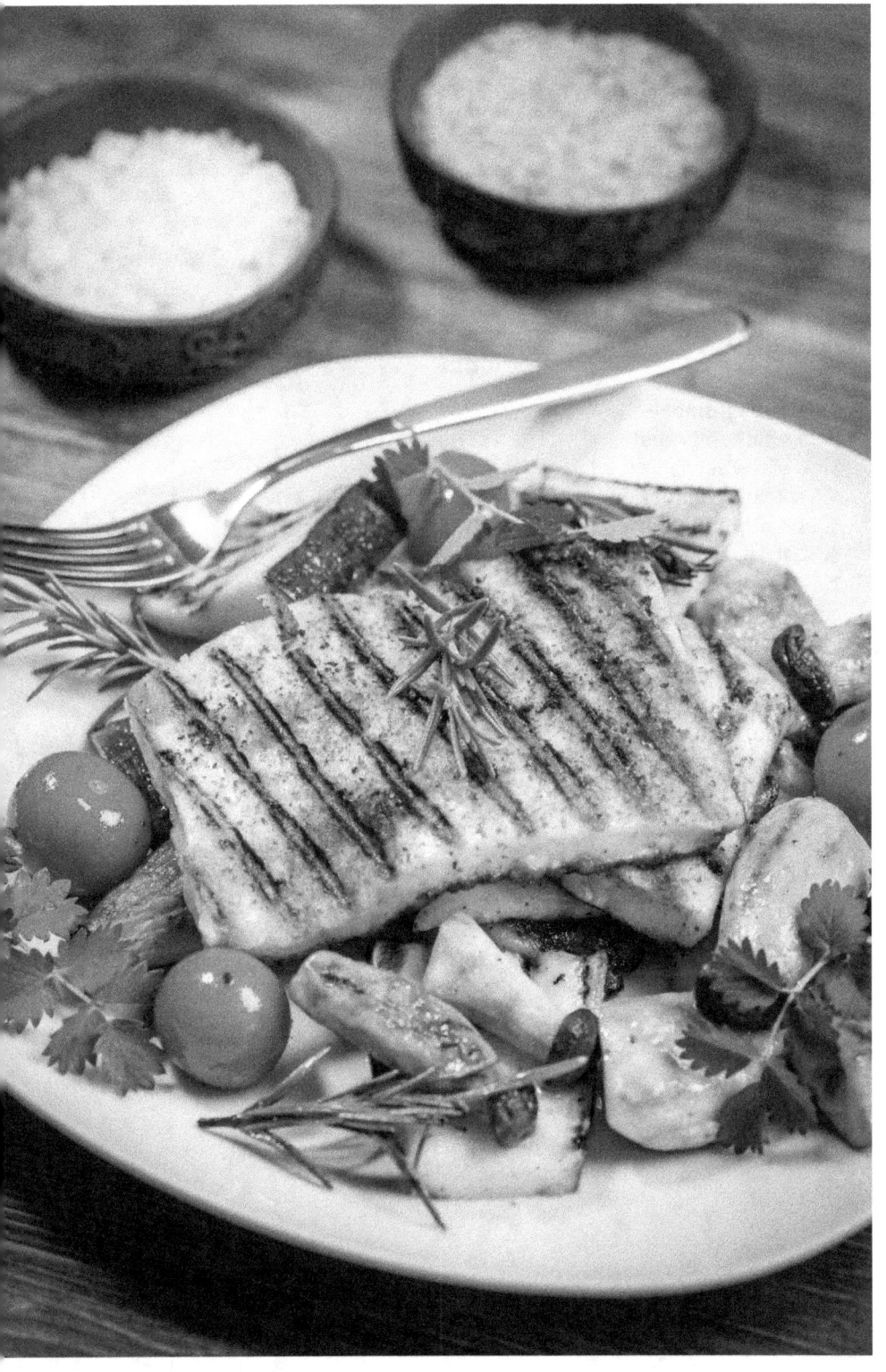

34. Chicken & Berry Summer Salad

Preparation 10 minutes

Calories 335

Fat 19g

Protein 21g

Carbohydrates 16g

Ingredients

1. 2 cups spinach
2. 1 chicken breast
3. 6 strawberries diced
4. 1/2 cup walnuts chopped
5. 3/4 cup blueberries
6. 3 tbsp. of raspberry balsamic vinegar
7. 3 tbsp. of feta cheese

Instructions

1. Slice the chicken breast into cubes. Cook in a pan. Set the cooked chicken aside to cool end off.
2. Chop, dice and then crumble your ingredients using a deep bowl and sprinkle your dressing on them.
3. Throw in your chicken and the dressing and toss!

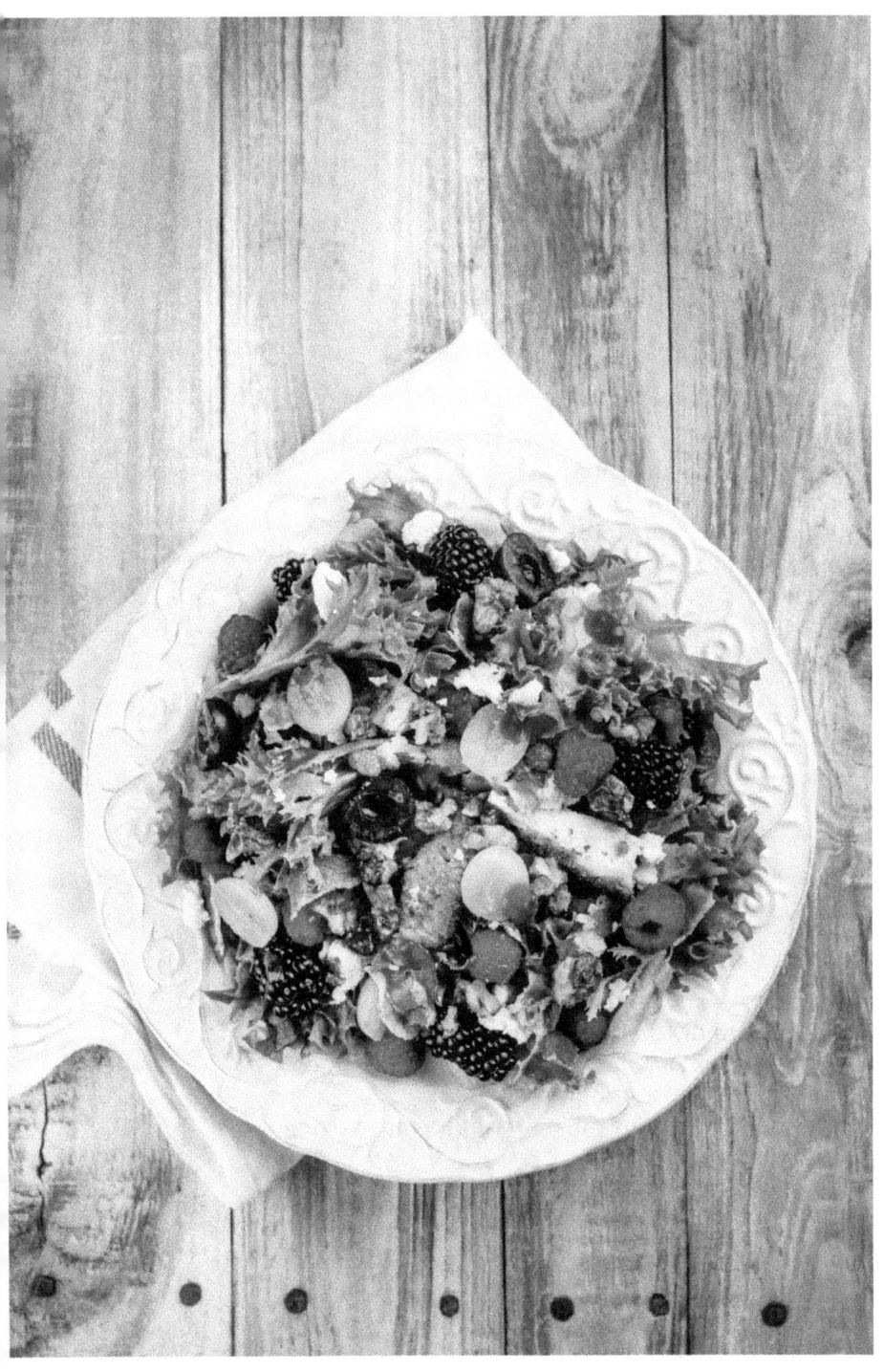

35. Keto tuna salad with poached eggs

Preparation time 15 minutes

Calories 765

Carbohydrates 6 g

Fat 69 g

Protein 29 g

Ingredients

1. 120 g tuna
2. Tuna Salad
3. 1⁄3 cup celery stalks, chopped
4. ½ red onion
5. 1 teaspoon Dijon mustard
6. ½ cup mayonnaise
7. Salt and pepper
8. 2 tbsp small capers
9. ½ lemon, zest, and juice
10. 60 g leafy greens
11. 60 g cherry tomatoes
12. Poached eggs
13. 2 tablespoons of olive oil
14. 4 eggs
15. 2 teaspoons of white vinegar 5%
16. 1 teaspoon salt

Instructions

1. Mix drained tuna with other ingredients for salad, except tomatoes and lettuce.
2. Bring water to the boil. Add vinegar and salt.
3. Stir water in circles and create a swirl with a spoon.
4. Crack egg into the stirring water.
5. Let it simmer for about 3 minutes and remove using a slotted spoon.
6. Drizzle olive oil before serving.

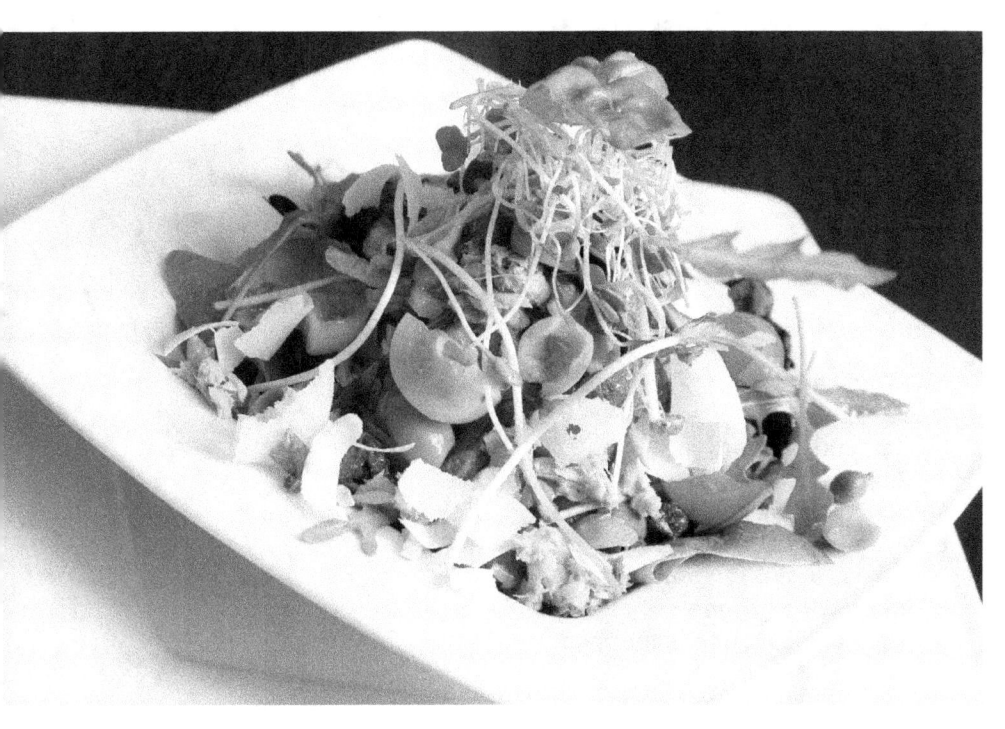

36. Warm keto kale salad

Preparation time 15 minutes

Calories 498

Carbohydrates 5 g

Fat 49 g

Protein 10 g

Ingredients

1. 220 g kale
2. 60 g butter
3. Salt and pepper
4. 2 tablespoons mayonnaise
5. ¾ cup of heavy whipping cream
6. 2 tablespoons olive oil
7. 1 teaspoon Dijon mustard
8. 120 g blue cheese
9. 1 garlic clove, finely chopped

Instructions

1. Mix mayonnaise, heavy cream, mustard, garlic, and olive oil in a beaker. Add pepper and salt.
2. Rinse your kale and slice into small pieces. Remove and throw away the thick stem.
3. Heat up a frying pan and add butter. Kale quickly to give it a nice color. Add salt and pepper.
4. Place mix in salad bowl and put the dressing on the top. Stir and serve you are your crumbled blue cheese.

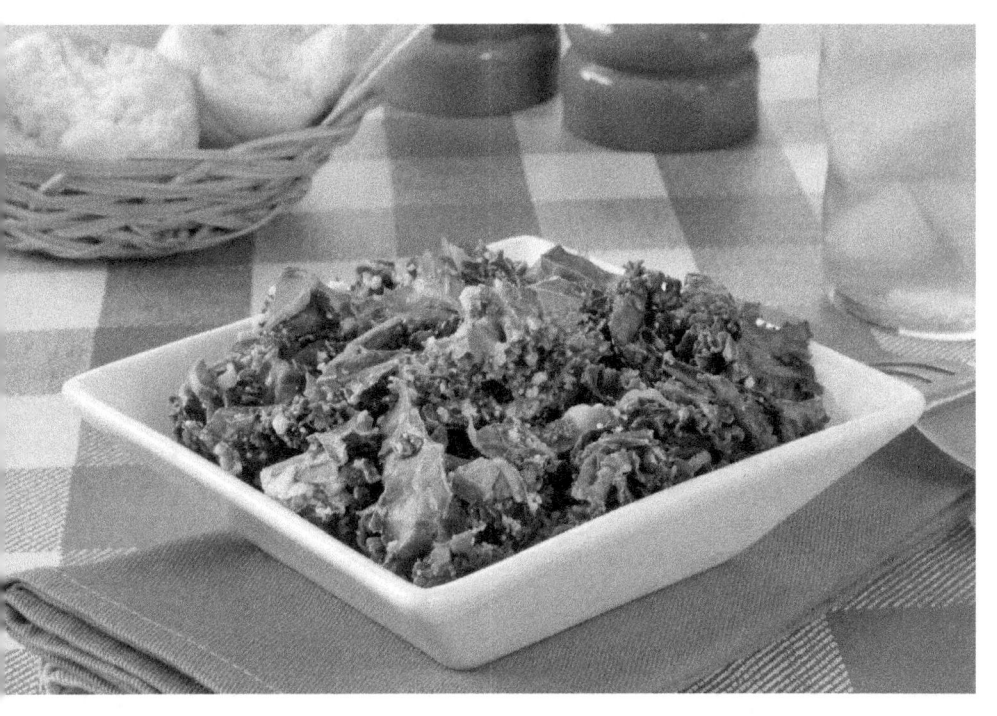

37. Grilled eggplant salad

Preparation time 15 minutes

Calories 444

Carbs 9 g

Fat 37 g

Protein 15 g

Ingredients

1. ½ cup olive oil
2. 800 g eggplant
3. ½ lemon, juiced
4. 200 g tomatoes
5. 100 g of fresh mozzarella cheese
6. 50 g anchovies
7. Salt and pepper
8. 4 tablespoons fresh mint

Instructions

1. Slice the eggplant and brush it with olive oil on each side. Add salt.
2. Grill until the slices are brown and really soft. Turn often.
3. Mix lemon juice, olive oil, and the freshly minced garlic.
4. Place the dressing on a dish and put the eggplant slices on the top to soak. Turn after a minute.
5. Slice the tomatoes and add to dish. Place anchovies over eggplant slices. Add sliced mozzarella and arrange them on top.
6. Drizzle some olive oil, drops of vinegar and lemon juice and season with fresh mint, and freshly ground black pepper.

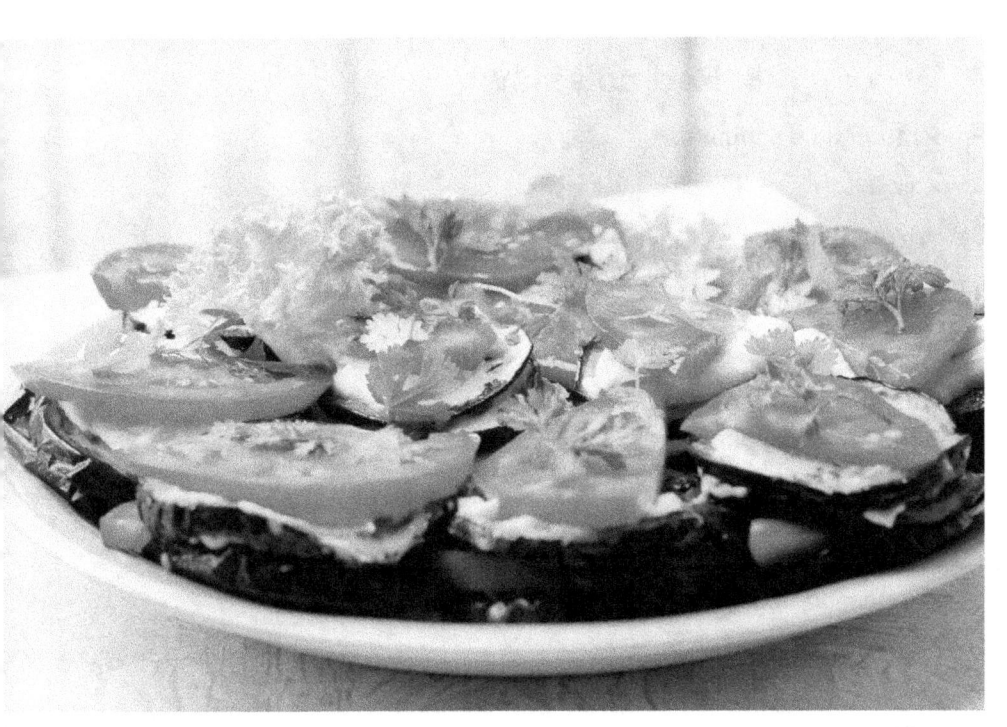

38. Red coleslaw

Preparation time 5 minutes

Calories 356

Carbohydrates 7 g

Fat 35 g

Protein 2 g

Ingredients

1. 1¼ cups mayonnaise
2. 250 g red cabbage
3. 1 teaspoon salt
4. 1 tablespoon of whole-grain mustard
5. 2 tsp of ground caraway seeds
6. ¼ teaspoon of ground black pepper

Instructions

1. Use a mandolin slicer and shred the cabbage.
2. Mix with the other ingredients and leave for 10–15 minutes and then serve.

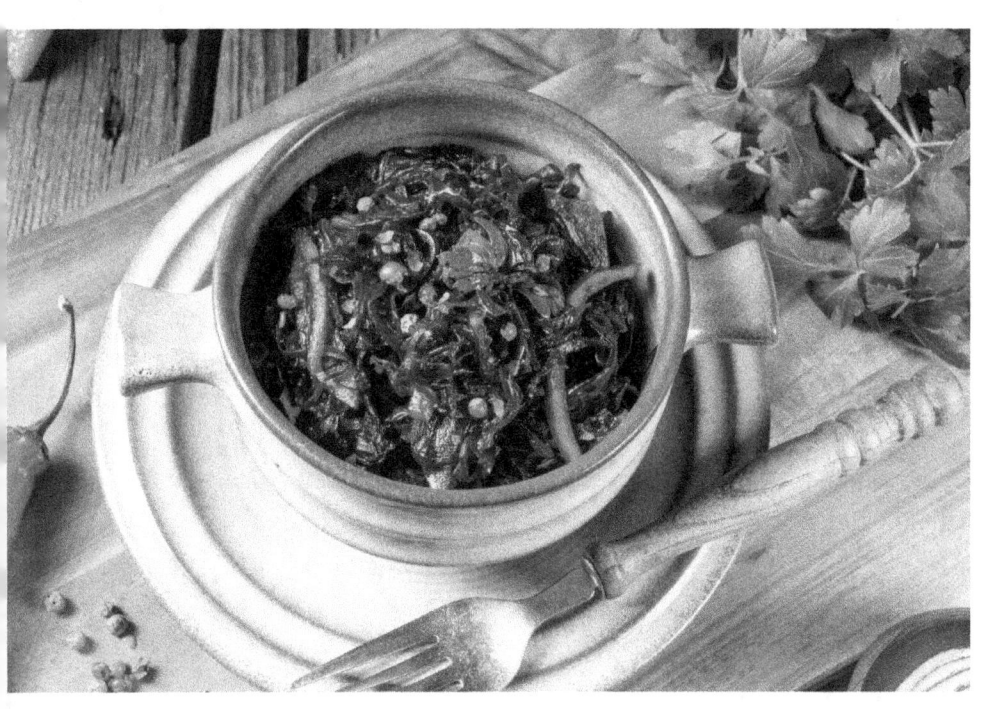

39. Eggplant salad

Preparation time 20 minutes

Calories 188

Carbohydrates 8 g

Fat 15 g

Protein 3 g

Ingredients

1. 2 green bell peppers
2. 2 eggplant
3. ½ cup fresh parsley
4. 1 red chili pepper
5. ½ cup mayonnaise
6. 1 lemon, juice
7. 2 garlic cloves
8. 1 teaspoon salt

Instructions

1. Preheat oven to 480ºF.
2. Cut the bell peppers and eggplants in half length-wise.
Seed the bell peppers.
3. Put the vegetables in an ovenproof platter.
4. Set the platter in the middle part of the oven, and bake
for thirty minutes, turn the eggplants after about twenty minutes.
5. Remove dish from oven and let cool.
6. Slice the chili and seed it.
7. Chop the chili finely.
8. Cut the parsley and pound the garlic.
9. Mix all with lemon juice in a bowl.
10. Remove the skins of the grilled vegetables. Cut them into tiny
dices and add to the mayonnaise and parsley mix.
11. Mix thoroughly.
12. Store for a few hours so the flavors can develop.

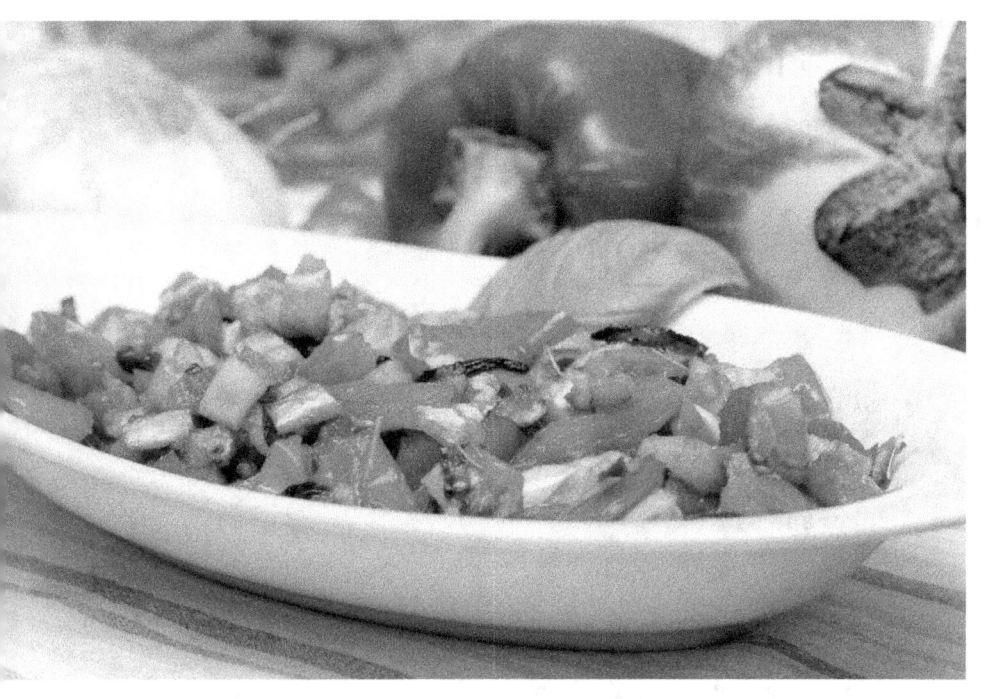

40. Caprice snack

Preparation time 5 minutes

Calories 216

Carbohydrates 3 g

Fat 16 g

Protein 13 g

Ingredients

1. 8 oz. mozzarella
2. 8 oz. cherry tomatoes
3. 2 tablespoons of green pesto
4. Pepper and salt

Instructions

1. Slice the mozzarella balls and tomatoes in half.
 Add the pesto and stir.
2. Add salt and pepper as desired.

Shopping list for ketogenic salad

Salad Mix

Spinach

Cauliflower

Asparagus

Celery

Cucumber

Broccoli

Green Beans

Eggplant

Limes

Mushrooms

Peppers

Lemons

Spaghetti Squash

Zucchini

Kale

Squash

Dairy products

Eggs

Butter

Sour Cream

Heavy Whipping Cream

Blue Cheese

Shredded Mozzarella

Ricotta Cheese

Shredded Cheddar

Cream Cheese

Swiss Cheese

All full-fat cheese

Parmesan Cheese

Fruits

Strawberries

Blueberries

Raspberries

Conclusion

Your keto diet can be spiced up with these tasty salad recipes. It doesn't have to be restrictive.

www.ingramcontent.com/pod-product-compliance
Lightning Source LLC
Chambersburg PA
CBHW071226220526
45468CB00002B/750